THE
200
CALORIE
SOLUTION

THE
200
CALORIE
SOLUTION

How to Burn an Extra 200 Calories a Day and Stop Dieting

MARTIN KATAHN Ph.D

Drawings by Melinda Pate

W · W · *Norton & Company · New York · London*

THE TEXT OF THIS BOOK is composed in photocomposition Baskerville. Display type is set in Delphian Open and Helvetica Bold. Composition and manufacturing are by the Maple-Vail Book Manufacturing Group. Book design is by Marjorie J. Flock.

Library of Congress Cataloging in Publication Data
Katahn, Martin.
   The 200-calorie solution.   Bibliography: p.
   1. Reducing—Psychological aspects.   2. Reducing
diets.   3. Reducing exercises.   I. Title:
II. Title: Two hundred calorie solution.
RM222.22.K345   1982   613.7'1   81–18808
                                       AACR2
W. W. Norton & Company, Inc. 500 Fifth Avenue, New York, N.Y. 10110
W. W. Norton & Company Ltd. 37 Great Russell Street, London WC1B 3NU

2 3 4 5 6 7 8 9 0

ISBN 0-393-01530-0

To Ruth and Rae
eighty plus and
walking strong

CONTENTS

INTRODUCTION

I am writing this book because, frankly, I am sick and tired of the garbage being written that touts dieting as a means for permanent weight control. Dieting to lose weight and continual dieting to keep one's weight down may work in five out of one hundred cases. And for those few people, long-term successful dieting usually means forever being deprived of one of life's great joys—good eating!

For most overweight people eating is a source of great pleasure. And if the way you choose to lose weight or to maintain desirable weight focuses on caloric restriction—calorie counting, protein powders, behavior modification—you are in for a life of semistarvation. In addition, the emotional effects are miserable. Since most dieters are always struggling, and frequently failing, they feel badly about their inability to control themselves. They take frequent "guilt trips" whenever they see the scale go up a couple of pounds after what they believed to be an episode of overeating.

Not only does dieting not work, but the latest scientific evidence proves that dieting actually makes it easier to gain weight! Each time you diet and then resume normal eating, you have a tendency to get even fatter than you were before. This fact, which I will explain, is grounded in the physiology and chemistry of your body.

If dieting is not the ultimate solution to your problem, then, what is? To answer that question, we have to ask first, "Why are *you* fat?" I am going to show you how to evaluate the cause in your own case in the first two chapters of this book, but I can already give you a tentative answer based on the latest research and informed scientific opinion: for most people less than fifty pounds overweight the *primary cause* is a sedentary lifestyle and not overeating. For people fifty pounds overweight or more, overeating plays a more important role, along with inactivity. *But the great majority of overweight Americans are not, in fact, eating more than the standards for people of average weight set by the Food and Nutrition Board of the National Research Council.* Indeed, according to a recent study of the United States Department of Agriculture, Americans are, on the average, eating considerably less than we did as a nation just a few years ago, *but we aren't losing weight.*

How can we eat less and not lose weight? The answer has to be obvious. We have compensated by becoming more and more sedentary in our daily habits.

Fortunately for the health of our nation there is a tremendous surge of interest in physical fitness. Walkers and joggers are beginning to crowd our streets and parks. But if you are overweight, you have probably just watched this boom in physical fitness benefit your thinner friends. Perhaps you have gone so far as to join a spa or buy a tennis racket—only to let your membership languish or your equipment gather dust in the closet.

Why is it that overweight, inactive men and women, the persons who can benefit most, are least likely to develop an active lifestyle— the *only* way to assure slimness and fitness?

Part of the answer is that overweight people do not fully appreciate the complex physical, psychological, and social forces that keep them fat. And even if they did understand these forces, most overweight people would not know how to go about changing them. Furthermore, our physical educators, physicians, nutritionists, and psychologists have not made a concerted effort to get the most reliable information before the public, nor have they developed specific approaches to fitness that would help fat people work toward their best body size or physical fitness level.

It is a pity, if not an outrage, that because of our nation's great interest in becoming slim, many unscrupulous people have entered the slimming business. These people often promise instant success for little effort, using miraculous secret diets or fat-burning pills (advertised appropriately on the back pages of the Sunday comics). Almost all the people seduced into using such approaches will ultimately be fatter than ever. Most of the ten billion dollars we invest annually in the effort to get thin is wasted, if not actually harmful to our health.

As a professional in the treatment of obesity and a research scientist in the area, I have tried to write this book in a way that will help you as much as if you worked with me personally. As you will discover, the approach is quite simple in concept. Once this method is implemented, formerly fat people find it hard to believe that they could have enjoyed any other kind of lifestyle and stayed fat. But, at the onset, it can involve making dramatic changes in the way you think, in the way you schedule your life, and in the way you relate to other people. It also involves developing the means to sustain your motivation through a long probationary period, during which you discover and cultivate some physical activity that will give you more pleasure than your former sedentary approach to living.

If you are more than a few pounds overweight, it will take sincere commitment to change your daily schedule, not only to include physical activity, but to include substitute activities for overeating. If you are *truly* an unwise overeater, you will need to develop new ways of thinking about food. I say *"truly* an unwise overeater" because, examined on a weekly or monthly basis, most overweight people are not eating an unreasonable amount. In fact, on the average, they do not eat more than thin people. I will show you how to determine the truth in your own case. But whatever the nature of your eating habits, you will have to learn to move your body in ways that make movement more enjoyable than painful.

By persistently following the approach I will describe, overweight people have lost 50, 75, even 125 pounds—and they are keeping them off. In contrast with other approaches, the unique benefit of the program is that your persistence will pay off in a way that may sound unbelievable to you today. Instead of being in danger of regaining weight, if you follow my approach, you will find it *harder to change back into the fat person you once were than it seems now to become thin and vigorous, even if you have been fat for years.*

Among my primary objectives in writing this book is to present an approach to fitness that has a higher likelihood of working for fat people, more than any other approach I know. Even in the best of circumstances and with people of average weight, fitness programs have a dropout rate of between 40 and 65 percent. However, as many as 90 percent of all fat people will drop out. In fact, percentage of body fat is the best predictor of who will finish an exercise program.

Fat people drop out of even the best-led exercise programs for many reasons. In part, because most exercise classes and conditioning programs are led by people who have never been fat and have valued fitness all of their lives. They have no idea what it is like to have grown up in a fat body and never to have acquired athletic skills. I grew up in a fat body, so I know. I was fifty pounds overweight at twelve years of age, and headed still upward. During the Second World War a fitness program was instituted at our high school. I could not do a single push-up or sit-up and scored lowest among over one thousand boys in the initial fitness test. I stayed seventy pounds overweight until the age of thirty-five. But then, with a combination of sensible eating and activity, I took off all of my excess pounds, never to put them back. I took up tennis, and became a competitive tournament player. I became a runner and bicycler at age fifty. From personal experience I know what it takes to overcome the many psychological and physical barriers to fitness that an overweight, embarrassed adult faces.

During the last five years I have pursued the subject of fitness in countless classes and workshops. I have put my understanding of psychology and fitness together in the process of directing the Vanderbilt University Weight Management Program in which over 1500 people have participated. Out of this experience, I have developed an approach to permanent weight reduction through the development of an active lifestyle which I believe is ideally suited to the temperament and physiological characteristics of overweight individuals.

The approach includes yogic stretching to increase flexibility and basic strength training to increase muscular endurance, both of which will decrease your chances of injury and help mold a body that moves with strength, grace, and agility. But, most important, the program hinges on activity that increases cardiovascular endurance, which, in turn, contributes to a higher energy level and to an overall sense of well-being. One incidental additional benefit of the overall approach is an increase in basal metabolic rate. Not only will you come to enjoy burning up the calories that would otherwise be stored as body fat, but you will have the pleasure of knowing that you are burning more of them just sitting still.

I will outline the physiological and psychological principles; I will present a program you can do on your own; and I will bring you to the point where you will be proud to join any fitness class, get out on the tennis court or dance floor, or jog through the park. You will be ready to undertake more advanced fitness routines usually reserved for teen-agers, if you so desire. I'll show you what to look for and how to get the best out of any supervised fitness or activity class, or how to add variety to your program completely on your own. And, if you *really* need to, I'll show you how to learn to eat sensibly as well.

ACKNOWLEDGMENTS

This book could not have been written without the encouragement and collaboration of many people.

I want to express my appreciation to my associates and former associates in the Vanderbilt Weight Management Program for the countless contributions they have made to my understanding of obesity and the development of an effective treatment program: Drs. John Pleas, Kenneth Wallston, Gordon Kaplan, Larry Weitz, and Faye Walter. My present graduate students, Ruth Daby, Mark McMinn, and Michael Thackrey, have made significant contributions with their diligent search of the research literature and the analysis of outcome data.

My colleagues in the field of nutrition and physical fitness have contributed greatly to my knowledge in their areas of expertise. They include Dr. Lee Fleshood and Ms. Mary Buckner, M.A., R.D., Director and Assistant Director of the Division of Nutrition, Tennessee Department of Public Health; Ms. Dorothy Bevington, R.D., Nutrition Consultant to the Vanderbilt University Weight Management Program; and Kent Rea, Southeastern Region Health and Physical Education Consultant and Associate General Executive of the Nashville Young Men's Christian Association. I also deeply appreciate their critical reading of my manuscript and their many excellent comments and suggestions.

Over the years many people have added to the file of recipes in the Katahn household, sampled our own cooking, and made creative suggestions. I have included some of these recipes in this book and want to give special thanks to my friends and colleagues Dr. Richard Blanton, Jane Wert, and Mary Buckner once again.

Ever since the start of the Vanderbilt Weight Management Program, many people who have enjoyed and profited from weight management and fitness groups under my leadership have encouraged me to write down my ideas and experiences, and to put my personal approach into a form that anyone could use without having to join a professionally supervised program. This book would not have been written, however, were it not for the constant urging of one person in particular, Ms. Barbara Pinson, writer and law student at Vanderbilt University. After participating in one of my fitness classes, losing twenty pounds and discovering the joys of long distance running, she convinced me that with a book it was possible to inspire other people to do what she had done, and that I could, in spite of my own doubts, write such a book. I am indebted to her for her criticisms of the first draft of this manuscript.

I want to thank Pat Burns for working so many long hours typing the manuscript and being helpful far beyond the call of duty.

To Enid, my wife of thirty years, I will be forever indebted for loving me as a fat man, marrying me and being a constant companion, and then collaborating with me whole-heartedly when I decided to lose seventy pounds and incorporate into my daily life the activities that have kept me slim, fit, and happy these last eighteen years. I am also indebted to her for her collaboration in our culinary experiments and for taking time from her own busy schedule of concerts and teaching to read and comment on the manuscript.

I feel especially fortunate in having Arthur and Richard Pine as my literary agents. Their personal interest in my work and enthusiastic help with all of those publishing details for which I have neither talent nor understanding are deeply appreciated.

Finally, I want to thank Star Lawrence, my editor, for the help I received while preparing the final version for publication. It's been a pleasure working with him and his staff at W. W. Norton.

THE
200
CALORIE
SOLUTION

I

200 CALORIES AWAY

Evaluating Your Activity Level

You are just 200 calories a day away from being permanently slimmer, healthier, and more totally alive. But, it is not counting these calories that does it for you—you must burn them! Let me give you the background.

Most overweight people in this country do not fully appreciate how inactive they are. They do not play physically active games. Many of them have never cultivated the basic skills to engage in sports. Technological advances have reduced the amount of movement and strength required in our daily jobs. About half the population in the country does not expend energy much above the resting metabolic level for a major part of their lives. The more inactive we become, the fatter. And the fatter we get, the less active.

Odds are that you are like the many overweight people research has shown to engage in fewer than two miles a day of walking. That is, you may be moving about on your feet for fewer than forty minutes of your entire waking hours. Many overweight people spend twenty-two hours or more every day either sitting or lying down, not even standing. Do you doubt this in your own case? Buy a pedometer and find out for yourself; count the time you spend standing or moving about. You will be impressed if not appalled. (I discuss pedometers in chapter eight.)

Thin people move considerably more on the average than fat people. In the same occupations, thin persons will move two to three miles a day *more* than their fat counterparts, but even this amount of activity compares poorly with that of our forebears. At the turn of the century, the average American was walking seven or eight miles a day. Unwittingly, Henry Ford may be more responsible for the epidemic of obesity in this country than any other single person.

Even in games and exercise, fat people conserve energy. Fat tennis players seem to have longer arms. Films confirm the relative lack of movement of fat adolescents during play. I remember a volley ball game with a group of overweight participants. The overweight folks might take a step toward the ball, but if they missed or made an error, it was our thin staff assistants who raced about, chasing and bending to retrieve the ball to put it back in play. The thin folks were getting all the exercise, and they didn't want to slow the pace and intensity of the game to match that of the fatter, slower participants. In a study of campers in our national parks, I found that the obese use equipment that requires less work, such as mobile homes rather than tents or tent trailers.

How much energy does an average person expend in a day? In 1980, the Food and Nutrition Board of the National Research Council estimated that the average woman twenty-three to fifty years of age weighing 128 pounds expended approximately 2000 calories per day, while the average man at 154 pounds expended 2700. Naturally, if you expend 2000 or 2700 calories per day, then, on the average, *you have to eat that many calories to maintain your weight.*

What does it take in the way of body movement, in addition to normal basal and resting metabolic requirements, to actually burn that number of calories each day? If we assume eight hours of sleeping, and nine hours of sitting and sitting tasks (which require approximately 1000 to 1100 calories for a woman of average weight and body fat, and around 1300 to 1400 calories for a man) it would take:

Five hours *of involvement in tasks combining standing and a small amount of walking about, or, standing in place with considerable arm movement, the equivalent of brushing teeth, washing dishes, making beds, unpacking groceries, arranging merchandise,*

PLUS

two hours *of moderate to brisk walking, approximately six miles at a three-mile-per-hour pace, or other work equivalent in energy expenditure. Work like bricklaying, carpentry, garage mechanics, mopping floors, raking leaves generally uses* slightly less energy *than continuous walking at a three-mile-per hour pace.*

Do not kid yourself. The average American comes nowhere close to doing this amount of activity. If you keep an honest record, you will probably find that you spend only about two hours a day in standing tasks, and one hour or less of actual walking, in any twenty-four-hour period.

And this is why the average American is fat. *We are, frankly, not active enough to eat like normal human beings!* Even our average-weight citizens have reduced their activity levels, but they are evidently also compensating, according to the Department of Agriculture, by eating about 10–15 percent less than they did at the time the Food and Nutrition Board gathered its data. A 10–15 percent reduction in calorie requirements actually means that many of us, certainly the overweight and sedentary, are spending less than two hours a day in standing tasks and one hour a day in walking, or its energy equivalent. Our bodies are marvelously adaptive to the demands we place on them. If we sit twelve to fourteen hours a day, what do we need? A fat ass! That's what we get.

Overweight people do not need nearly the number of calories per day in food that standard nutritional texts recommend for so-called sedentary or light-activity lifestyles. Daily caloric requirements for women of average weight in sedentary occupations are estimated at fourteen calories per pound of body weight, while in light activity, women are said to need around sixteen calories per pound of body weight. Because they are larger and have more muscle mass, men may need approximately two calories more than women, or sixteen to eighteen calories per pound of body weight in sedentary or light-activity occupations. If your job involves sitting most of the day, it is sedentary (secretarial work, reading, and studying). If it involves standing *most* of the day, with moving about, it is light activity.

These caloric intake estimates are quite appropriate for persons of average weight, but they are not for the overweight. As we go up in weight, and as a larger percentage of our weight goes to fat, we need relatively fewer calories. We need fewer because fat tissue is relatively less active metabolically than other tissue, and sedentary fat people are *more* sedentary than thin people. They find ways to conserve movement in every occupation, and thus they burn fewer calories. As weight goes up and body fat increases, and as activity declines to that measly two miles of walking per day, women's caloric requirements become as low as ten calories per pound of body weight per day, and men may reach down to about twelve calories per pound of body weight. *Thus, many 200-pound women can, and do, eat only as much as their 128-pound counterparts. The same for many fat, inactive men of around 250 pounds. They are not eating any more than active males of 160–70 pounds body weight.*

What would it take in the way of extra activity to compensate for the sedentary lifestyle that is responsible for most cases of slight to moderate obesity? You must restore the equivalent of 200 calories of energy expenditure to your life each day.

The average overweight person is about three miles *short* each day of walking his or her way to permanent weight loss, better health, and a more attractive body. Put another way, about forty-five minutes a day of brisk activity would do it. It would take several hours of singles tennis or racquet ball each week, somewhat less of swimming and bicycling, and even less of jogging (but I do not recommend jogging for overweight people—certainly not at first).

So, evaluate yourself on this all-important activity dimension. First, buy a pedometer—adjust it carefully since most pedometers overestimate the distance walked. You will probably find that you walk less than five or six miles a day. If you don't wish to buy a pedometer, keep track of the number of hours you engage in walking activities. You will probably find that you walk less than two hours per day and very little of it at a brisk pace. Second, review the activity content of your average day. You are probably on your feet less than two hours, on the average. Third, total the extra physical activity that you spend in games and sports per week. It takes about five hours of active sports each week to compensate for a lifestyle that averages only two or three miles a day of walking and only two hours a day standing on one's feet performing other tasks.

I have titled this book *The 200-Calorie Solution* to emphasize that adding an average of 200 calories of energy expenditure to your life each day is a good guarantee that you will not regain whatever weight you lose following temporary, moderate caloric restriction, when you start to eat "normally" again. Our research results show that in one-, two-, and three-year follow-ups of people who initiated a weight loss campaign, virtually all who increased their daily energy expenditure by 200 calories have lost weight and kept it off—some twenty pounds, some forty pounds, and some considerably more. Very few people who try to lose weight by dieting alone can say that.

As I said, our bodies adapt marvelously to the demands we place on them. If you use more energy each day in tasks or games that are done better in a lighter, stronger body, then that is the kind of body you will get. Of course, a sound diet is basic to our health whether we are reducing or trying to maintain our weight. Most of us can improve our nutritional habits as I will recommend, and be healthier and feel better for it. But almost all people who try to lose weight by diet alone will not keep it off. In the following chapters where I discuss principles of sound nutrition and safe, sensible dieting, I also explain why low calorie dieting without a change in your activity level, only increases your fat building capacity. With sensible, high calorie dieting and *activity,* you can lose just as much weight as you can with fad diets and crash diets. In the beginning,

FIG. 1   *Relative importance of activity and dieting in permanent weight control.*

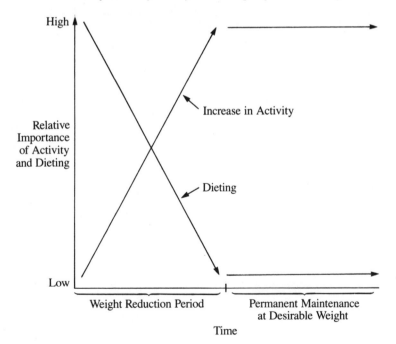

my Double Your Fat Loss Diet gives you the satisfaction of *safe, rapid* weight reduction. But, when you reach desirable weight, caloric restriction becomes far less important. For all but the grossly obese, an active lifestyle in and of itself is the ultimate fat solution.

Figure 1 illustrates the relative importance of dieting and increasing activity during the weight loss period itself, and then for maintenance at desirable weight. When you begin a weight loss effort, adherence to moderate caloric restriction is the key to a rapid initial loss. During this period, *you build your daily activity level.* As the weeks go by, activity takes over and becomes *the all-important ingredient for permanent success.* Persistent burning of an extra 200 calories* a day in forty-five minutes of walking, or other equivalent physical activity, means you can *stop dieting* and eat like a normal human being after you reach your goal weight.

Keep the diagram in Figure 1 firmly in your mind's eye as you begin your activity program, and watch the pounds and inches come off.

---

*This activity usually has the additional effect of changing basal metabolism so that you *burn 100 to 200 more calories* during the other twenty-three or so hours of the day.

2

DO YOU REALLY HAVE
AN EATING PROBLEM?

"How do I know I eat too much? I'm fat, aren't I?"

When I ask this question of prospective patients, I invariably get that answer, so ingrained is the notion that obesity is caused by an unreasonable amount of eating.

But, is it? Take a look at this menu. It contains three meals from different fast-food chains. I have selected these meals because we usually think of them as highly caloric.

BREAKFAST
Grapefruit juice, hot cakes with butter and syrup, tea or coffee
512 calories*

LUNCH
Hamburger, order of french fries, medium-size cola drink
542 calories*

DINNER
Fried chicken dinner: three pieces of chicken, mashed potatoes and gravy, cole slaw, roll, and medium cola drink
930 calories*
Total **1984** calories

This menu is loaded with starch and foods high in fat and sugar. As continuous daily fare it would be deficient in many of the vitamins, minerals and dietary fiber the body needs, *but it won't make*

*Calorie count taken from information supplied for standard servings by McDonald's, Burger King, and Kentucky Fried Chicken.

the average woman who follows my program of reasonable daily activity fat.
A reasonably active man could add a couple of slices of bread and
butter, another piece of fried chicken, and even a piece of apple
pie. This would *not* be a healthy diet, *but he would not gain weight.*

Let's take a look at a more nutritious "high calorie" day of eating. I have arranged this menu by food groups in order to make
some additional points.

	CALORIES
MILK	
2 cups low fat milk (1 percent fat)	204
MEAT	
3½ ozs. roasted or broiled chicken, light meat only	166
3½ ozs. canned pink salmon	141
FRUITS / VEGETABLES	
½ cup orange juice	56
3½ ozs. (¾ cup) fresh pineapple	52
½ cup carrots	26
⅔ cup broccoli	22
GRAINS	
3 slices whole wheat bread	168
1 cup puffed wheat	50
	Subtotal 885
FAT	
3 teaspoons butter (as bread spread or flavoring)	108
OTHER	
2 twelve-ounce colas	258
2 oz. fudge	224
2 cake doughnuts	250
1 piece (3½ ozs.) custard pie	200
	Grand total 1925

This diet pattern, without the added fat and the other foods
listed, at only 885 calories,* approximates the intake of essential
nutrients suggested by the National Research Council (NRC) Com-

*Calorie values based on Pennington, Jean A. T. and Church, Helen Nichols. *Food
Values of Portions Commonly Used.* New York: Harper & Row, 1980.

mittee on Recommended Dietary Allowances (RDA). If you choose
your food from each of the four groups listed, but vary the meats,
fruits and vegetables, and grains each day, you would not be likely
to suffer any nutritional deficiency on a short-term basis and you
would lose a great amount of weight. Dieting this severely, however, is not necessary and not good for you. I developed this sample menu, including the "fat" and "other" categories, to emphasize
two points.

1. Adding to a basically sound, low-calorie diet two colas, two
pieces of fudge, two cake doughnuts, and even a piece of custard
pie—really fattening foods, right?—*is not going to make the average
woman fat if she follows the activity program I recommend.*

And men, because of higher caloric needs, could add more meat,
bread, and pie than I have already included in this very ample
menu and not get fat.

2. Once you get active by simply restoring forty-five minutes of
physical activity to your daily life, *you will be able to stop dieting.* There
is room for fat and carbohydrates in the active person's diet.

Of course, when I speak about sound nutrition, I am not going
to recommend eating exactly the menus in these examples. But,
think back over your daily food intake this past month. Do you, on
the average, eat more than I have included in these two sample
menus? It is a rare person who does (unless you are fifty pounds
or more overweight). And so, my guess is that you do not either.
The problem lies elsewhere.

Being Scientific about Calorie Needs

Most people can make a good guess about the extent to which
overeating may be the culprit in their weight problem from the
above discussion. But they remain incredulous. They can't believe
that they ought to be able to eat as much as I suggest. They still
cannot accept the idea that anything but their eating habits can
cause their obesity.

Because you, too, may remain skeptical I want to explain the
cause of obesity from the scientific standpoint, using the concept of
energy balance. You may already have read about this concept, but
chances are you have overlooked its key implications.

1. To maintain a given weight, the calories in the food you eat
must, over time, equal the calories you burn maintaining bodily

functions (your basal metabolic rate) and the additional calories you burn at work and play.

2. At a reasonable level of physical activity (a level appropriate for the average American and one that is demonstrably conducive to good physical and mental health) the average woman of 128 pounds will use approximately 2000 calories per day. A man of 154 pounds needs about 2700. These are exactly the amounts illustrated by my "high calorie" menus.

3. Most overweight people in this country *do not* eat more than these suggested amounts. A great many are eating considerably less.

4. But most overweight people in this country never engage in any activity that gets their metabolisms up above their resting levels. They rarely walk more than a few blocks at a time; they rarely play active games. Thus, over an extended period of time, *just by eating normally,* they have accumulated an excess of fat.

5. *Once a person has become fat, a normal intake of food is used to maintain the larger sedentary body.* Both an active woman of 128 pounds and an inactive woman of 200 pounds can eat the same amount of food each day. The first never gains weight; the second stays fat.

Thus, as long as you are not eating more than the amounts I have mentioned, I do not consider you to have an eating problem as far as calories are concerned. You have simply upset the energy balance. You have put calories that daily moderate activity would have burned up into your fat stores. We are going to reverse that process. The concept of energy balance explains how today you may be a woman of 200 pounds, eating 2000 calories, and how in the near future you can be at ideal weight and still eat the amount you do today. The same 2000 calories necessary to maintain the 200-pound body in the sitting position are necessary to maintain the 128-pound body that spends more time in the walking position.

I know that many of my readers will say to themselves, "This doesn't apply to me. I'm not average. My metabolism is slower than normal. I'll never be able to eat like that."

I am particularly concerned about women who entertain this thought. Certain popular writers are spreading the idea that all fat women have abnormal metabolic processes that require them to follow low calorie diets for the rest of their lives. Don't believe it!

This is dangerous. Low calorie dieting and a lack of activity are exactly the things that make your body adept at storing fat. It's the fallacious remedy itself—on-again-off-again, low calorie dieting—that may actually be causing you to get fatter and fatter.

I want to assure you at the onset: even if your metabolic rate is slower than average, you can compensate, and, at least to some extent, raise it, by eating as I advise and becoming active. You will prove it to yourself. You may end up needing 20 percent, possibly 30 percent, more calories each day living slim than you do now as an overweight person. I know from personal experience. Many formerly fat men and women really do eat, as I do, more now that we are slim and active than we did when we were as much as seventy pounds heavier.

If you have any concern about slow metabolism, I will show you in chapter twelve how to verify your personal caloric needs, how to predict and control your weight loss, and how to determine what you can eat to maintain yourself permanently at ideal weight.

Eating Nutritiously

Although the great majority of overweight people are not consuming too many calories, *an overwhelming number are not eating wisely.* This goes for thin people, too. I know from my research with both overweight patients and college students of average weight: only one in five persons in these two populations consumes a diet that comes close to meeting 100 percent of the Recommended Dietary Allowances (RDAs) suggested by the NRC Committee. Fortunately, the NRC standards are set so high that most people will not show obvious signs of nutritional deficiencies even when their diets approach only 75 percent of the RDAs.

Nevertheless, I believe that certain psychological symptoms are associated with a combination of this borderline nutritional status and lack of physical activity. These symptoms can include fatigue, irritability, and mild depression on the one hand, or restlessness and insomnia on the other. Assuming no illness or severe trauma, I relate these symptoms to diet and the sedentary lifestyle because they almost always disappear when people change their eating and activity habits. Even though I'm convinced that diet plays an independent role in these symptoms because digestive processes work so much better when you eat right, I cannot pinpoint the relative contribution of diet and inactivity to these psychological problems because people who follow my program change many aspects of their lifestyles in addition to their eating habits.

When my nutritionist associates and I do a detailed dietary analysis, we have people keep careful eating records for several weeks. They are taught to weigh and measure food portions. We can evaluate nutritional status by calculating the amounts of all the nutrients generally present in the foods they have eaten.

But such record keeping is a very tedious process. Over the years I have found that the answer to *one* simple question can tell me almost as much as an intensive dietary history. Answer it for yourself. Think back over the past several days:

Do you, on the average each day, eat more servings of fruits and vegetables combined than you do of fried foods, fat saturated snacks (like potato or corn chips), desserts, soft drinks, and candy combined?

If the answer is "No," I can predict with a great deal of certainty that (1) whether you are overweight or not, your diet will be too high in fat, and possibly sugar, foods; (2) if overeating, as well as inactivity, is indeed contributing to your weight problem, it will usually be because you eat too much fat and possibly too much sugar; (3) your diet may be borderline with respect to vitamins A and C; and (4) you are not making a conscious effort to eat nutritiously and your diet will probably be borderline in other respects, e.g., dietary fiber, calcium, iron, and B vitamins.

Yes, all of these things usually show up when we do a more detailed analysis.

If you eat fewer servings of fruits and vegetables than you do of junk foods, you are definitely not eating wisely. You will get a better idea of where you may be lacking when you complete the following checklist.

A Dietary Checklist for You and Your Family

Nutritionists advise us to think in terms of four food groups as we select our food each day:

    I. Milk and milk products (primarily for calcium, riboflavin, and protein).

    II. Fruits and vegetables (primarily for vitamins A and C, and fiber).

III. Whole grains (primarily for complex carbohydrates, iron, B vitamins and fiber).

IV. Meat, fowl, fish, and certain plant alternates (primarily for protein, iron, and B vitamins).

Assuming variety, if we have two standard-sized servings from the milk group, four of fruits and vegetables, four of grain products, and two of meat, fish, or fowl each day, we may obtain approximately 1200 calories from these sources and come close to the RDAs of all nutrients. We may still, however, be short on calcium, iron, and some B vitamins.

It doesn't matter whether you eat southern style, Italian style, or Chinese style. Because the average woman who follows my program is able to eat approximately 2000 calories a day and men 2700, there is room for some added fat (for cooking and flavoring), moderate amounts of alcohol if you desire, some dessert, and other snack foods.

Fancy recipes are fine. As long as a variety of foods within the four groups is represented in the diet in the minimal amounts specified—and it's only about 1200 calories worth in a diet that can include 2000 to 2700 calories—then you can be fairly sure that you are obtaining a large percentage of essential nutrients.

Although standard nutritional recommendations are "adequate," even these can be improved upon. In chapter ten, when you begin to use my Double Your Fat Loss Diet, I will make simple suggestions for permanent changes in your eating habits that will keep your energy level high and minimize any tendencies to store fat. My recommendations reflect the very latest information relating to sound nutrition.

But for now, let's just see if the eating habits of you and your family are adequate. Keep the following checklist as you continue to read and prepare to begin the program. Do one for yourself. If you have children, do one for each of them. Work out one for the family based on the meals eaten at home, and let the other family members fill in the record for meals eaten away from home. See whether the habits your children are developing are conducive to good health, and determine whether food preparation and service in the home is furthering sound nutritional practices. If unwise eating habits are in truth playing a role in your own obesity, you may be unwittingly setting the stage for a similar problem in your children. I don't think you want to do that.

Dietary Checklist
Section A

Food	Credits	1	2	3	4	5	6	7
Milk and other calcium sources: (cheddar cheese, 1.5 oz.; milk, yogurt, 1 cup; salmon, sardines, 3 oz.; cottage cheese, 2 cups)								
one serving	15							
two servings	15							
(children must have three servings, adolescents four, to earn 30 points in this group)								
Fruits and vegetables:								
one serving, green or yellow vegetables (½ cup cooked, 1 cup raw)	10							
one serving citrus fruit, tomato, cabbage, green pepper (portions commonly served)	10							
two or more servings other fruits, vegetables, potato	10							
Breads and cereals:								
at least four servings of whole grain or enriched cereals (see package for serving size) or bread (1 slice per serving)	15							
Meat and other protein sources:								
1–2 eggs, one serving (2–3 oz.) meat, fish, poultry, cheese,*; (or 1 cup dried beans or peas),	15							
one or more additional servings	10							
Total								

*Count cheese as milk *OR* meat, *NOT* both simultaneously.

DIETARY CHECKLIST

Section B

Enter a checkmark [√] for each serving, OR for any food in Section A that was fried

Food	Day 1	2	3	4	5	6	7
Dessert							
Soft drinks							
Alcohol							
Candy							
Fried food							
High-fat snack (potato or corn chips, etc.)							
Total √s							

Instructions for Weekly Checklist

Section A Give yourself the credits indicated for each serving of food from each of the four food categories. Children require one additional milk serving to earn thirty credits from calcium-rich food sources. Adolescents should have two additional servings. The fruit and vegetable credits have been allocated to help assure adequate sources of vitamins A and C, and fiber. I reluctantly include enriched bread and flour foods with whole grain products in the bread and cereal category. Many nutrients are lost in the milling of grain that are not replaced with enrichment programs. If you eat a wide variety of other foods, you can compensate for this loss. But more and more nutritionists are urging us to return to whole grains in our diets. I compare the value of whole grains versus enriched flour in table two in chapter ten.

A score of 100 on this section of the checklist helps assure your meeting the RDAs of essential nutrients, with the possible exception of iron, at a calorie intake of between 1200 and 1400 calories. Obviously you can have additional servings of foods in these four categories to meet additional calorie needs. If you choose more food from these four categories, you will be increasing the nutritional value of your diet. However, you can also select dessert, drinks, and other foods as indicated in Section B of the checklist to meet additional energy needs.

Section B Enter a checkmark any time a food listed in section B is eaten, or any time something in section A is prepared by frying. If you score *below* 100 in section A and have *any* checks here, your diet may be lacking in the essentials, and you have substituted relatively empty calories to meet your daily energy needs.

If you score 100 in section A, and have three or more checks in section B, watch out. While fried foods that qualify for credit in section A and some desserts do contain essential vitamins and minerals, and your score of 100 does indicate that you are probably meeting essential nutritional requirements, *you are also taking in a large amount of fat and/or sugar or alcohol.* Active people can burn up a large amount of calories from these sources (even though it would be much better for them to obtain their additional energy in a more nutritious manner). For fat people, however, these calories serve little purpose other than to maintain extra large fat stores.

If you are like my students and my overweight patients, I think you will be impressed at the results of this record. Eighty percent of the people I have tested score less than 100 in section A, and have three or more checks in section B. If this turns out to be true of you, I think you also will be impressed with how much better you feel when you engage my program and change some of these unwise, if not fattening, eating habits.

Psychological Aspects of Eating

Most people who come to me for help believe, like everyone else, that eating is the cause of their obesity. Because I'm a psychologist, they expect help in breaking bad eating habits and in understanding the psychological causes of their supposed eating problem. Indeed, sometimes bad habits and emotional problems do play a role, especially in severe obesity. Fortunately, these cases are in a minority.

The critical factor as far as weight is concerned is whether an average of forty-five minutes of activity each day is going to be enough to compensate for any bad habits or emotionally driven eating behavior. If it is, it then becomes a matter of choice whether a person wants to change in these respects. *It is not essential.*

Let's examine the bad eating habit notion first. Because behavioral psychologists believe that obesity is an eating problem, they plunge in with a massive attack on the cues in the environment that are associated with eating. They also instruct patients on how to change their eating style. We are supposed to eat in one place only, dissociate food from the TV set, slow down our pace of eating, and so on, over a wide range of change strategies. If overating is in fact a problem, these strategies can be helpful. But first, we have to prove the case that overeating *is* the problem.

My point is that it usually isn't. Both fat and thin people eat in front of the TV. Many of us, both fat and thin, eat relatively fast. If underactivity is the problem, as the majority of overweight people discover when they evaluate their activity levels as I have suggested, it's treating the wrong end of the horse to attempt to make permanent (unrealistic and unnecessary) changes in eating habits. It's still the old dieting approach dressed up in new clothes.

As long as your food intake is not over 2000 to 2700 calories (depending primarily on whether you are female or male) the easiest and most enjoyable solution to the obesity problem is to change your activity level. You can still eat fast—even do it in front of the TV. That is not where the problem lies.

The conclusion is similar with respect to the emotions and eating behavior. Although the emotions can play a decidedly important role in a few cases, usually in severe obesity, it causes needless additional stress among most fat people to spread the notion that eating in response to tension, anxiety, anger, or boredom is at the root of their problem. Compared with the amount of overeating caused by negative emotions, I believe far more needless tension is generated among fat people by encouraging them to diet continuously as a means of weight control.

Considering cultural influences and our biological make-up, fat people need to understand, without guilt, that it is perfectly natural to eat when we want to celebrate and to feel relaxed after a meal. Food is a natural accompaniment to a festive occasion. And with respect to tension, all animals become quieter after eating. Because food brings down our arousal level, some people have learned to use eating to reduce tension, whatever its cause. But, emotional eating leads to weight problems only when caloric intake becomes higher than reasonable activity can burn off.

Notwithstanding all these facts, fat people still feel that the eating and emotion association is bad even if it isn't a cause of their obesity. And this is where my program has some of its most beneficial effects.

First, increasing your activity level makes you feel more energetic and elevates your mood throughout the day.

Second, increased activity is a great antidote for tension, both normal and extreme. For those instances where tension truly drives a person to overeat or drink, the substitution of a walk, jog, or tennis match for an eating binge or a double martini, serves a triple purpose. It decreases calorie intake, increases calorie expenditure, and acts as a more enduring tension reducer than eating or drinking.

Third, the lifestyle changes involved in the development of activity are themselves the best antidotes for boredom and the irritability and depression that frequently go with it. In addition to becoming an enjoyable physical experience in its own right, the process of developing an active lifestyle leads people into new social circles. New friends frequently enrich the quality of life.

Fourth, and most important for those in whom emotional factors do play a causative role in obesity, the development of an active lifestyle does wonders for the self-concept and self-control. Active people come to like themselves better. And in the process of becoming active, people gain psychological as well as physical strength. You may have doubts about your willpower when it comes to food today. You won't in the future.

So, for the time being, let's reserve judgment on the role poor eating habits and other psychological issues may play in your weight problem. If these prove to be important in your particular case, I devote chapter eleven to teaching you how to cope with them.

3

WHY ACTIVITY SUCCEEDS
WHERE DIETING FAILS

Have you ever noticed with dismay how easy it is to regain weight right after you've dieted? The day you get off your diet, it's whammo—three pounds up, then up and up on much less food than it took to keep you fat in the first place.

I have already explained why dieting is an irrational approach when the major factor that contributes to obesity is inactivity. There are yet additional reasons why dieting is a disaster.

Repeated or prolonged low calorie dieting makes it easier and easier to get fatter and fatter on less and less food.

It breaks my heart to talk to people—the majority of them women in their thirties and forties—who, with repeated dieting and sedentary lifestyles, have trained their bodies to get along on 1500 calories per day and sometimes even less. Their misguided physicians still hand them 800-to-1000-calorie diets. Once or twice a year they embark on the newest miracle diet that promises "as much as twenty pounds off in fourteen days." Some starve themselves completely for a week at a time. A few have gone into hospital wards and fasted for months.

Have you tried one of these really low calorie reducing plans? Where is your weight now? The more drastic the approach you used, the heavier you are likely to be today.

It's time you understood the facts and stopped this self-defeating, insane dieting behavior.

Here is what happens to your body when you go on any low calorie diet without changing your physical activity level. (I consider anything below 1200 calories for a woman and 1500 calories for a man too low and almost always unnecessary when weight reduction is approached correctly.)

1. There is an immediate, large water loss. Although the average weight loss on diets of 1000 calories or less can approximate five pounds in three days, only a small fraction of the loss is body fat. In the first week of such a diet, more than 70 percent of the load off your scale can be the result of water depletion.

2. Your body begins to burn protein, which is normally used to maintain cellular structure and strength. One consequence is that you begin to lose muscle mass.

3. *Your body interprets severe caloric restriction as a threat to life itself, and marshals all its defensive forces:*

a) Fat cells show biochemical changes in an effort to maintain their size and retain fat.

b) Hormones and enzymes involved in energy production are produced in lower quantities.

4. As a result of these defensive reactions, body metabolism slows down. Within a matter of days it will slow anywhere from 10 to 45 percent. This means that you begin to use 10 to 45 percent fewer calories keeping your vital functions going (your blood circulating, brain and body organs working, and body cells repaired and regenerated). In some ways, the slowing of metabolism is like turning down the thermostat in your house. Work goes on but you learn to do it in an atmosphere that uses less fuel.

Ninety-five percent of dieters now experience the following reactions, all of which are determined, at least in part, by physiological and biochemical changes:

1. Within two weeks, weight loss slows dramatically. Then you start to hit plateaus and sometimes suffer inexplicable sudden gains of one to three pounds.

2. Within a short time you may notice a lack of energy. Going up a flight or two of stairs can exhaust you. Your endurance for sustained activity is gone. You suffer "downers" in the late afternoon.

3. You may be hit with more frequent headaches and periods of irritability. If you have any predisposition to constipation, the condition frequently gets worse.

4. Your initial enthusiasm for the diet begins to wane. The first

five to ten pounds were pretty easy, but now you are going at a snail's pace. Between the social pressures to resume your normal eating practices and your own desire to eat as a normal human being, you decide to have just one regular meal. You think to yourself, "I'll go back on the diet tomorrow."

5. But your weight doesn't hold steady after one regular meal. Instead, you gain at least a pound—more likely two or three. And it all won't come off the next day, or sometimes even the next, even though you are back on your diet.

6. You find it harder and harder to be letter-perfect with your diet. You start to "half-diet." *But even though you are not eating as much as you did before the diet, your weight is slowly creeping back up.*

Unbeknown to you, your body is playing a nasty trick and sabotaging your effort. *This is happening because you have chosen an unhealthy way to lose weight.*

Here is what is going on:

A dramatic slowdown in weight loss occurs when you have finally gotten rid of all of the water your body can spare from its tissues, especially that part which was stored in your muscle cells and liver. In the first few days of a diet you burn up a large part of your quick energy stores—the sugar, in the form of glycogen, that is stored in the liver and muscle cells. In a normal day's activity, about half the energy you use is supplied by glucose (the form of sugar to which glycogen or the carbohydrate in your food is transformed when you need it for energy). The other half of the energy you use comes from fat.

Because you are dieting and not taking in your usual amount of carbohydrate for energy, your body is required to burn the stores in the liver and muscles. Here is the important fact for weight losers: glycogen is stored in a solution of water, *about one part glycogen to between three and four parts water.* Remember that ratio.

You may have about one pound of glycogen (2000 calories or a little more) that can be depleted from your liver and muscle stores. With it will go almost four times its weight in water. This is the source of a major part of the body's water loss, which is in turn the major part of your entire weight loss in the first days of a diet. Another part of the water loss is due to the lower amount of sodium contained in your reduced caloric intake. If you have chosen a low calorie high protein diet, you will also lose significant additional amounts of water. Your kidneys work extra hard to rid your body of toxic byproducts produced by the metabolism of your own body protein as well as the large amount of dietary protein now burned for energy rather than for repairing and regenerating body tissue.

Once you have rid yourself of this large amount of water and the rate of weight loss has slowed, you are susceptible to plateaus and seemingly inexplicable weight gains from anything that can affect your water balance. One of my patients demonstrated that a single bowl of onion soup can lead to a full three-pound weight-gain. The first time it happened she could not believe it, so we repeated the meal that led to the gain a week later. That convinced her. A single bowl of onion soup may have the sodium equivalent of a full teaspoon of salt. Another patient, in the early days of my obesity work when I recommended high protein diets, ate a sweet potato (without butter, mind you) and a single chocolate chip cookie. In a low carbohydrate diet, that amount of extra carbohydrate acts just like sodium in the body. She gained over two pounds on that splurge of about 250 surplus calories. Even when a person goes right back on a diet, it can take as many as three days to lose all that water—and if you don't get right back to work and only "half-diet," within a week or two the water weight will in reality be replaced by fat weight.

The loss of energy that people often experience on diets is primarily the result of the depletion of energy stores in the liver and muscles, the lowered production of hormones and enzymes used to put glucose to work, and the burning of muscle tissue protein. Glucose is especially important as an energy source at the onset of any movement (getting up from a chair), or in any movement that is so strenuous it is difficult to continue for more than a few minutes. Climbing stairs or carrying a heavy load of groceries are everyday examples of more strenuous work. Sedentary, overweight people find these activities quickly tiring even when they are not dieting because their muscles have not been trained to store large quantities of glycogen. A diet depletes them still further.

Add to the glycogen depletion the fact that the body starts to convert protein stores to energy and you have an actual reduction in the size and strength of the muscles you need to perform your daily tasks. Besides weakening you, this will slow your metabolism slightly, since you are losing active tissue.

For many people the headaches and irritability that accompany the severe disruption of bodily function caused by dieting are transitory. If you stick to a very low calorie diet long enough, you may even experience a kind of euphoria that occurs as people face death from starvation. One thing that does not disappear for many dieters, however, is the problem of constipation. Low calorie diets, especially the high protein varieties again in vogue, do not provide the body with the necessary fiber to keep intestinal functions flowing smoothly. Dosing with bran helps some, but it is dangerous for others. They end up with diarrhea and inflammation of the lower intestine. These latter misfortunes were also experienced by many individuals who were persuaded to experiment with the Beverly Hills Diet.

If you manage to get beyond two weeks of dieting, you are faced with that drastically reduced rate of weight loss. There are three reasons for this.

First, you are now burning your fat stores, but for every gram of fat burned you lose far less weight than you did for every gram of stored sugar that you burned the first two weeks and, you must do nine calories worth of work to burn a gram of fat, but only four calories to burn a gram of your sugar stores.

Now, recall my mentioning that sugar is stored in the body with water in a ratio of about one part sugar to three or four parts water.

Fat is stored in a ratio of from two to three parts fat to only one part water.*

If you burn three-quarters of a pound (almost 1500 calories) of your sugar stores in week one, you will lose roughly three more pounds in water. Together, that's a three-and-three-quarter-pound weight loss. If you also burned 1500 of fat, you would have lost almost another one-half pound. Total: four and a quarter pounds for a 3000 calorie restriction.

What do you get for a 3000 calorie cutback in week three or four? Because the glycogen pool is depleted and that large amount of water is gone, you lose, in the main, only the weight associated with fat: about one pound if you're lucky. No wonder the dieter gets discouraged.

---

*These figures cannot be made more precise because the ratio can vary among tissue sites and from person to person.

The second factor affecting weight loss is a tendency to reduce already low activity levels still further. Low calorie diets, especially the unbalanced fad diets, reduce your energy level and your endurance so much that you tend to avoid any unnecessary movement. A reduction in activity is a natural reaction as your body tries to match energy outgo to the reduced intake.

But by far the most important self-defeating effect of dieting has to do with your metabolic rate.

The more drastic your diet, the more likely your body will undertake drastic countermeasures. Body metabolism slows as much as 45 percent. This reaction is so important that I want to give you a detailed illustration of its consequences.

Most women weighing as much as two hundred pounds do not eat 2000 calories a day. I continually repeat this point because 2000 calories is a reasonable intake, *but many overweight women have trained their bodies to get along on considerably less through inactivity and repeated dieting.* They have also trained their bodies to defend against the onslaught of each new diet by increasing their ability to *cut back quickly* on metabolic needs.

This is what occurs all too often for a woman of around 200 pounds trying to reach ideal weight on a diet of 1000 calories or less. Whereas at sixty to seventy pounds overweight she may have needed 2000 calories to maintain herself, within days after beginning the new diet, her calorie needs start to fall. If her needs fall as much as 40 percent, she will be expending only 1200 calories in her daily activity instead of 2000. Assume she is a good dieter and sticks religiously to 1000 calories per day: if her body had continued to need 2000 calories she would be saving 1000 calories each day. She would be losing weight at a reasonable clip—an average of about two pounds per week. But she doesn't need that many calories anymore. She is down to a 1200 calorie requirement. The thousand calorie diet provides her with a true saving of only 200 calories per day—or 1400 calories *per week*. She will be lucky to average a half-pound weight loss each week for the rest of her diet.

Every diet book I've ever seen that has been written for the layman, including some by otherwise knowledgeable health professionals, states that if you reduce your food intake 3500 calories you will lose a pound of fat. *This is simply not true. You must reduce your energy intake 3500 calories below your actual energy expenditure to lose a pound.* No wonder it's frustrating when your body reduces its energy expenditure 40 percent. You are cutting back 1000 calories per day, but your body is compensating for—wiping out—800 calories of your heroic effort. Sounds a little like gross inflation when your dietary restriction of 1000 calories is, in reality, worth only 200 calories of weight loss. In the *average* person, the decrease in metabolism will generally range between 15 and 25 percent. However, the more obese the person, the more extreme the diet, and the greater the frequency of low calorie dieting in the past, the greater the probability that the slowdown will exceed that range.

The story has not ended. So far, so bad—but the worst is yet to come.

By slowing your metabolism you make it easier to gain weight on fewer calories than it took to maintain yourself before you began to diet. Whereas it may have taken 2000 calories to maintain your prediet weight, now you can start to gain it back at only 1300 or 1400 because your body has cut its needs down to 1200. As you regain your weight, your body tries to readjust to your previous caloric needs, but it may not make it all the way back to the full requirement of 2000 calories. So, if you resume eating at the 2000-calorie level, you will probably gain at least several extra pounds over your prediet weight. Even worse, because your body was doing everything it could to maintain its fat storage while you were dieting, it learned to increase its ability to conserve fat. There is every likelihood that a greater overall percentage of your new weight will be fat. If you weighed 200 pounds before you dieted and had 40 percent body fat content, you may soon hit 210 pounds and have 45 percent body fat.

Now you have the physiological facts on which I base my admonition to fat people:

Never go on a diet to lose weight.

That is, not unless you are willing to change your activity level. In order for a diet to work once and for all, you must remove the critical contribution of a sedentary lifestyle to your weight problem. Then you will never need to diet again.

So far I have been speaking theoretically. Let me give you an actual example from an incident that took place after I had made a presentation of my views before the employees of a large industrial organization that was interested in starting a weight management program. A young woman raised her hand and commented that she disagreed with what I had said, especially that part about being able to eat 2000 calories a day and losing weight on a 1200-calorie diet. She had personal experience to prove I was wrong.

She said that about ten years ago when she was approximately thirty-five pounds overweight, her doctor put her on an 800-calorie diet. She lost down to the vicinity of her present weight—130 pounds. At five feet three inches tall, she still feels she is about ten pounds over her ideal weight. However, she finds that she cannot eat anywhere near 2000 calories and she cannot lose weight efficiently on anything more than 800 calories.

How did she know that? On the basis of what she felt were accurate eating records that she had kept for her doctor on many occasions during these past ten years.

Here is her history in brief. She has used that 800-calorie diet on the advice of her physician three to four times a year. When she is not dieting, she claims she gains about ten pounds over a three-to four-month period eating an average of only 1600 calories. Then it's back on the diet. After the first three-to-four-pound water loss, she claims she can only lose a pound a week on 800 calories and nothing at all on 1200.

I told her I was impressed with her ability to diet so faithfully, but I asked her if she did anything in the way of physical activity or had combined diet with exercise in order to lose weight. The answer was negative. No time—long hours of work, and a husband and young children to care for at home were her reasons.

I restrained myself from uttering the first thought that came to my mind. "No wonder you can't eat 2000 calories and can't lose weight on 1200." Instead I told her she was evidently correct about herself, but for the very reasons I had just talked about. My analysis is as follows:

1. Losing a pound a week on 800 calories per day indicates that she is eating about 500 calories a day below her actual energy needs. While dieting, her true energy expenditure is about 1300 calories. A daily 500-calorie deficit between energy intake and energy expenditure does add up to that 3500 calories required for a weekly weight loss of about a pound.

2. She regains weight on 1600 calories—possibly averaging a half

pound a week, after that first three or four pounds that goes with putting the glycogen store back—because she only needs 1300 when she gets off her diet.

3. Then, by the time her caloric needs readjust from 1300 calories upward to her nondieting level several weeks down the road, she has most of her ten pounds back.

4. As a supertrained fat conserver because of her repeated dieting and sedentary lifestyle she is quite correct: right now she cannot eat 2000 calories and she cannot lose on 1200.

But I could not have had a better example to prove the points I had tried to make in my speech. Just forty-five minutes of some sort of physical activity and she could climb off her yo-yo once and for all.

Activity Means Success

In contrast to the effects of dieting, here is what an active lifestyle contributes to weight loss and maintenance:

1. Activity can compensate for any metabolic slowdown that occurs during the sensible, temporary, high calorie dieting I recommend.

2. Even if your metabolism is on the slow side, activity can *forever* compensate for as much as a 20 to 30 percent variation.

3. Combining activity with diet, both energy level and endurance will remain high, provided you use the principles I outline in my Double Your Fat Loss Diet.

4. Activity can prevent the loss of muscle mass. This keeps your strength up and helps elevate your basal metabolic rate.

5. Activity requires that a higher percentage of the energy content of your food flow into your muscles and liver storage system. It reduces the amount that needs to be placed in fat cells after eating, to be withdrawn between meals. More energy is used for muscle cell maintenance, less for fat cell maintanance.

6. This alters your biochemistry. At both hormone and enzyme levels, changes take place to facilitate the utilization of energy through activity and reduce the ability to store fat and maintain large fat deposits.

7. In very sedentary, severely obese people, who may have true eating problems, a faulty relationship of food intake to energy

expenditure is rebalanced through activity. In some cases, moderate activity reduces appetite. It frequently strengthens one's motivation to stick to a temporary diet.

8. The body adapts itself in every possible way to your new lifestyle. In addition to the biochemical changes I mentioned above, your cardiovascular system increases in endurance, making activity feel easier all of the time. Even your bones change in composition—they become less brittle. In fact, one of the best ways to prevent the bone deterioration that accompanies aging, including that brought about by the hormone changes in menopause, as well as by the burden of carrying too much weight, is to stay active.

Here is a perfect textbook example of the importance of activity in weight control. A nutritionist colleague lost thirty pounds over a six-month period through a combination of diet and increased activity. Her activity consisted of a two- to three-mile walk (thirty to forty-five minutes) with her husband each evening after dinner. She maintained her weight loss for a period of a year and a half until both she and her husband changed jobs and discontinued their walking. Then, over a three-month period, she gained five pounds. When we discussed what had happened, she swore that she had not changed her eating habits. In order to understand better the cause of her weight gain, she started to keep an eating and activity record, using a pedometer to gauge her walking behavior. Over the next three months she gained an additional five pounds, but true to her claim, she was still eating reasonably at approximately 1800 calories per day. Her pedometer, however, showed a daily average of slightly less than two and a half miles. By discontinuing her evening walk, she had cut her energy expenditure approximately 200 calories a day. Her energy balance was thus displaced 200 calories on the intake side: 1800 in, only 1600 out.* This is almost exactly the amount it takes to gain ten pounds over a six-month period: 180 days × 200 surplus calories a day = 36,000 calories.

At about 3500 calories per pound, her gain can be explained by the decrease in energy expenditure when she stopped walking.

* At 57 years of age and 160 pounds, 1600 calories per day is about all any sedentary woman will need because metabolism slows with age (see table, chapter twelve). With a walk each evening she could have been eating 1800 and not gained.

This demonstration convinced her to get back on the track and start walking again.

Activity is your insurance policy. In my discussion and examples I have illustrated how dieting is the surest way to increase your ability to get fat and to stay fat. Dieting will not work unless you are willing to continually deprive or repeatedly starve yourself. I have also described how activity encourages your body to develop all its hidden potential right down to the cellular level for getting thin and staying thin. Just 200 calories a day expended in walking or its equivalent will keep at least twenty pounds of fat off your body each year.

Now I want to show you how getting active can give you more pleasure than just about anything you have ever done in your life.

4

THE MENTAL PART OF GETTING ACTIVE

The more sedentary your present life, the greater your surprise will be at the ultimate pleasure an active lifestyle can bring.

But making changes is not always easy. If you have already made an unsuccessful effort to get active, you know the difficulties. You have a right to be skeptical about my promise that I can show you a way to make it easier and more satisfying than your previous attempts. You know much too well that social pressures, work and family responsibilities, and the inertia of the body at rest can all combine to frustrate your best intentions.

I have learned a great deal about what it takes to fight the forces that work against permanent change from follow-up interviews with long-term successful weight losers. I think you, too, will learn from these stories and be inspired by them in the way my patients are.

Here is an example of what it takes for many women in the housewife and mother roles:

I had to argue with my husband just to get one evening off to come to the group meeting. Maybe it was my own fault, in a way, because he believed that men did such and such, and women such and such. And I went along with it. I was a fulltime mommy and I used to believe that mommies did everything around the house and everything for the kids. Whatever my husband wanted to do, well, that was a man's way—it's his right.

I was getting irritable. I knew it was mainly the way I looked. I was twenty-six years old. I had children, two and five, and I love them. Housework is okay, too, but I had put on twenty-five pounds since I got married, and I was beginning to hate myself. I was getting irritable and crabby all of the time, and I knew it was what was happening to my body. I am pretty short, and the twenty-five pounds made me look dumpy. I was looking ten years older and I was beginning to drag around like an old lady.

I finally decided to do something about it. I really had to fight at first. And, you know, I was always afraid to rock the boat—I always had to keep the peace—I always needed to keep things smooth. I think I was afraid I'd lose him if I got angry. But finally I made up my mind and boy, he objected at first. In the end I said "Okay—Okay, you're tired when you get home. I'll make dinner before I go to the group. I'll clean up. I'll get the kids ready for bed. You put them to bed, okay? Surely you can do *that much!*"

Well, he agreed, even though he kept a mad face on the first couple of weeks on the nights I went out. So, I started learning how to control the things that made me eat wrong—and I discovered walking! I must admit I used to think walking was so unglamorous. It didn't seem to be exciting like jogging. But when I get out there early in the morning moving along in a brisk stride, it's, well, I don't have to tell you, do I?—it's really invigorating.

The best thing about it is my conversations with myself. I don't tell anyone about this—but you asked. I like to talk to myself. I have imaginary conversations with other people sometimes. You know, what I should have said, or what I'm going to say—stuff like that. And now that I look so good—I really, *really* like the way I look—I think about the clothes I'm going to wear, or something I want to buy. I think about what I'll wear when I go to a party, or out to dinner. I think about what I'm going to say to so-and-so—you know—someone who's going to be there.

Sometimes I have real sexy fantasies. I'm not going to do anything really—I love my husband, and I'm not going to do anything to hurt my marriage—but I like to think about feeling sexy and being sexy. Maybe some people wouldn't like it, but I think it's okay, and boy, sometimes I really get going—you know, in my imagination.

Maybe it goes back to wanting to be a model when I was growing up. I knew I wasn't going to be one, but now, when I'm striding down the sidewalk, I want people to look at me. I want to show off, I want men to compliment me on how I look. Sometimes for a while, I'm a model—you know—my imagination—and I feel inside of me 'this is how a model walks.' I feel purposeful as I walk, but kind of sexy too. I'm not being provocative. I'm just feeling strong and beautiful.

And a lot has changed at home. I started hiring babysitters during the day so I can get out. I work a few hours a week—it pays the babysitters. I go to the Y for a dance class, and that is so much fun, and I'm not afraid to say what I think.

My husband is sharing a lot more things with the kids, too. I say "I'm going shopping. I'll take Karen with me. You keep Liz." And he says "Okay." He really likes me a whole lot more now that I'm independent and I say what I mean.

I have talked with many formerly fat people in an effort to find out what distinguishes the successful weight losers from the failures. I have interviewed people who did it on their own and others with the help of weight groups. Each story is unique, but common themes emerge. When I try to tell others how these people were successful, using their own words, I wish I were a poet, or at least more gifted as a writer. I would add to my presentation of their words something that would recreate the enthusiasm in their voices, the looks on their faces, all of the gestures and the spirit which help me feel, along with them, their own joy and wonder.

You may be asking yourself, "How does all of this relate to a fitness program for fat people?" Just this: a successful transition from a sedentary to an active lifestyle depends upon what happens in your mind. I suspect hundreds of books have been written on fitness—maybe thousands. They all concentrate on what you need to do with your body.

The authors of fitness books do attempt some mental manipulations, of course. They usually appear in the titles of the books, where you are led to believe that you can get fit instantly, or maybe in ten minutes a day, or, at most, in thirty minutes three times a week. But the exercise routines are still there. You find you have to move your body. You spend a few days trying to squeeze a routine into your schedule. You rush trying to get through with it as fast as you can. You are uncomfortable, and you may start to hurt. You do not see any immediate changes. Where is the pleasure and the success you have been promised?

The truth of the matter is that these approaches get you started on the wrong foot and with the wrong mental attitude. If a sedentary lifestyle is at the root of your obesity, an active lifestyle requires more than ten minutes a day, or three quick exercise sessions at the health club each week.

It takes forty to sixty minutes a day (I use forty-five minutes as a ballpark figure) of some kind of moderate physical activity to become, as Dr. William Glasser labeled it, "addicted." As I attempt to guide you into an active lifestyle, I'll try to communicate what is going on in the minds of people who are becoming addicted, or who have already made it.

A Decision for Fitness

You may have made as many resolutions to get fit as you have to diet. It only takes an instant to feel the urge to do something about your weight, but your decision must be renewed daily, until the feelings in your bones demand that you be active. That day will come. I assure you that persistence will transform you, so that a year or two from now you will not recognize yourself. The high point of your day will be your tennis match, your walk or jog, or your aerobics dance class.

But how do you get from here to there?

One of the first issues you will face is that of "finding time." Here is how Jean, a young woman, twenty-four years old and now forty-five pounds lighter, described how she went from square one—virtually zero—to a highly active lifestyle:

I had to face it—by using the "I'm so busy I don't have time to get active" excuse, I was saying that I had decided that *everything* else in my life, *every single thing,* was more important than losing weight and getting fit. And then I was feeling sorry for myself because I was so fat and wasn't having the kind of social life I wanted, and a lot of other things that kept me saying "I need to lose weight."

The first thing I realized was that I used to lie around in bed at least fifteen minutes after I woke up. So, I began to get out of bed sooner and started to do the "Good Morning" routine. I do the first stretches as I wait for the hot water in the bathroom. You remember how I hated to look at myself in the mirror? Now I do all of these exercises without any clothes on. I always turn sideways and look at myself in the mirror in the bathroom. I'm checking out my stomach. I say to myself each morning "Yep, my tummy is flat." I also get on the scale each day. I want to be glued to 110 pounds. [She is five feet three inches.] But I can vary two or three pounds up before I get excited about it.

Then I continue with my exercises, more stretching and a few strengthening exercises in the kitchen as I make coffee and breakfast. My whole morning routine takes between ten and fifteen minutes.

[I reminded Jean that I wanted to know about fitting exercise into a busy day.]

Well, I used to think I didn't have the time. I kept the daily log, and I wrote down for a week every single thing I did, just as you suggested. I found I had all the time in the world to fit in a walk, and you know, of course, I am running now. But it took willpower at first, until I found some other people to walk with and started making walking dates. Now I run with friends about half the time, and alone half the time.

[I asked her which she preferred.]

Both, really. It's equal. We talk when it's a social run, and when I'm alone, I see the world.

I knew what she meant about "seeing the world." Walkers and joggers discover a new relationship with their surroundings. Whether you walk or jog in the city, or along the countryside, your sense of your surroundings changes. You get a different feeling about the way you fit in the world, and discover a new sense of self. While it is indeed hard to describe, it can be experienced!

I can describe, however, the routine that Jean uses. I will also show you the simple strategy for getting your life in order so that there is plenty of time for your favorite activity. Because her social situation changed after she decided to place a priority on different behaviors in her own life, Jean now finds it perfectly natural to run three or four miles several times a week, take yoga classes, and even get to a health club three times a week for body conditioning. This new behavior is just as natural as it used to be to sit around and stay filled with fat and self-pity. She finds far more time, on the average, than forty-five minutes a day to do the things that make her look good and feel great. Whereas in the past she moved in a circle of sedentary friends, she now has a circle of active friends. Her social relationships provide the support for her new interest in activity.

Visions of Strength and Beauty

What keeps people going? What motivates people to beat those twenty-to-one odds against them, cut back temporarily on calories, and build their activity levels up to the point where they can then burn all the calories they'll ever want to eat? There is no way I want to deceive you about the problem! While some people easily lose ten pounds in two weeks, it can sometimes take ten to twelve weeks before you see and feel a real difference in physical condition. It can take as much as a year or two to become truly addicted to physical activity—addicted to the point that it becomes an essential ingredient of *your* new definition of a good life—and addicted to the point that it actually would be harder to go back to a fat way of living than it was to lose weight and get active in the first place.

We know that when people are asked, "Why do you want to lose weight?" they almost always answer with either a cosmetic or a health reason. Since so few succeed, we know that there must be some special ingredients in their motivation compared with that of the failures. Most people who analyze the situation think that those who succeed are just "more strongly motivated" than those who fail.

There is much more to it than that. It is not simply a matter of more or less, strong or weak, motivation.

Motivation has many components. You start with the desire to look better, maybe even to save your life. But unless some very significant psychological (and often social) changes take place, the new style of living and thinking that is essential to the weight loss period and then to weight maintenance will never win out over those well-established patterns that have kept you fat all of these years.

On the surface of it, you are motivated to lose weight. But you are also "motivated" to linger in bed, to work many long hours (because you have to) at a sedentary job, to watch television in the evening and on the weekends, perhaps to have a two-martini cocktail hour on the way home from work, or to raid the refrigerator from 5 P.M. until midnight. You are *not* motivated to walk or jog for forty to sixty minutes, or to play tennis or some other game every day. And you are not at all certain you're going to be motivated to try the program I am about to suggest.

What transpires in the minds and bodies of formerly fat people that makes the *process* of being thin more gratifying than the *process* of being fat? How does walking for forty-five minutes a day become one of the most satisfying, rewarding experiences of your existence, when, at this time you may not be able to walk six blocks without getting out of breath and without hating it? Obviously, something drastic must change inside of you, mentally and physically, if you are ever going to *enjoy* living the kind of life that coincidentally keeps you thin and fit!

I had never paid special attention to the key motivational components in my own success when I lost weight some eighteen years ago. The event took place thirteen years before I began to work in the obesity area. It took a number of follow-up interviews with successful weight losers to drive the point home to me, to make me fully aware of what had happened in my own case, and what was happening in theirs. Up until these interviews, I, like many other researchers and clinicians, had focused my attention on the overt behaviors necessary to weight loss, and not on the important inner processes.

It took one very special interview about three years ago with a young woman named Cindy, who had lost sixty-one pounds and kept them off for four years. It was she who showed me the magic of the mind and the importance of getting the mind and body to work together. Like most of us, she began with a cosmetic goal. But, along the way, a new relationship of thoughts, fantasies, and behaviors emerged that made it possible for her to reach that cosmetic goal.

I was going to be thirty years old. Each year I was getting fatter and fatter. I couldn't look at myself anymore. My boyfriend wasn't saying anything, but because I hated myself, I think it was my own feelings that were making sex less satisfying, and we just weren't doing it as much. I was ugly. I couldn't believe anyone would want to touch me!

[I had seen how Cindy looked before she lost weight, and she certainly was not ugly by any objective standard. But here is how she continued.]

One night I took off my clothes and forced myself to look in the mirror. I grabbed the fat around my hips and held it up in big blobs. I put my hands under my big fat belly and lifted it and shook it up and down so I could really see it. The fat was hanging down in folds. My skin was beginning to stretch and I was afraid that I'd never have a firm body again. I started to shake and I started to cry. I cried for a pretty long time. When I ran out of tears, I began to imagine what I might look like again—maybe—if I lost weight. I went over my body carefully—my legs, my belly, my breasts, my arms. I got a picture of the way I wanted to look again. Maybe, because I wasn't always fat, I saw the old me. I swore right then that I was going to do it and look like me again.

So, I got started. For almost a year, I carried every meal to work—no more snack foods. I cut out all desserts and junk. I started jumping rope and walking. I walked at every opportunity. I never sat down unless I had to. [Cindy wears a pedometer to this day, every day. By the end of the day it invariably reads between five to seven miles.] I watched how thin people moved. I wanted to move like that again. I wanted to feel and look like a feather. It was awful at first because it took so much effort.

[Cindy's next words and actions opened my eyes.]

I hit plateaus. I would go for two or three weeks and not lose an ounce. It happened more than once—I don't know how many times. I knew exactly what I had eaten. I had been perfect, absolutely perfect. And damn it, I wasn't losing weight! That's when I would get in front of the mirror again and take off all of my clothes.

[At this point she leaned forward and thrust her fist out at me with such ferocity that I startled and fell back several inches in my chair. With teeth clenched and shaking her fist, she growled:]

I would look at myself in the mirror and shake my fist at myself and say "I'm a fighter—*I am NEVER going to give up*. I ... am ... not ... a quitter! I am a FIGHTER!" I did this every time I felt I couldn't make it. It's funny, too, because I still do it in my imagination [the clenched fist]. Sometimes when I get into a tough situation, in my mind I just say to myself, "I am a fighter," and I never give up.

I thought about this interview for a long time. Cindy was so emotionally charged when she told me her story that it left me with my own heart racing. I began to compare the stories other successful people had told me and my own experience many years before.

All successful people, each in his or her own way, make dramatic changes in their mental processes. Cindy did two things. The first (which many of us have tried to do) was having a clear picture of the goal in her imagination—the way she wanted to look and the way she wanted to feel when she moved. The second, and probably the most important, was the image of herself as a FIGHTER. When she leaned forward in her chair, her whole body tensed and mobilized in that powerful gesture. I could feel the strength of her determination. When she assumed that posture, she was a warrior. This was the imagery that maintained her motivation through her most difficult days.

Fat people say to themselves and to others, "I do not have any willpower when it comes to eating and getting active." Then they behave in accordaince with that judgment of themselves. Not Cindy. Never again. Cindy is a fighter. When she makes that statement, she demonstrates with her body and her words that she has a will of steel. Then she acts in accordance with the self-concept of a fighter.

Cindy is a perfect example of what I mean when I say that when the mind and body work together, you can make it. You have to take the things you say to others, your fantasies, and all of the things you say to yourself, and then link them up with the things you do with your body. Being a fighter implies certain actions, and certain actions demonstrate that you are a fighter. Soon it becomes part of a single unified process: thoughts and actions become linked and express the new self-concept.

Cindy's rebirth as a thin person was quite dramatic, and there was considerable struggle in the accomplishment. In my own case something happened that made it relatively easy after thirty-five years of dieting failures. But I had to get hit over the head a few times. First a series of blood clots in my legs, and then what was diagosed as a mild coronary. From the age of twelve when I was fifty pounds overweight and had my first attack of thrombophlebitis, I had dieted on and off without success. Then, at the age of thirty-five, the coronary incident. I had just moved to Nashville and my new doctor was ahead of his time. In addition to suggesting a diet, he ordered me to get active.

In my childhood I had an uncle whom I idolized. He was an outstanding tennis player of national caliber. But he wouldn't even show me how to hold a tennis racquet! There was no way, in his mind I am sure, that such a fat, sloppy kid like me, fifty pounds overweight at twelve years of age, could ever be a tennis player. But a week after I got that advice from my doctor, I was on the tennis court in my street clothes with a borrowed tennis racquet. I found I could hit the ball and even though I was exhausted in half an hour, my childhood dream of being a tennis player was kindled anew. I was out on the tennis court again a few days later. Soon I started lessons, and soon I was playing every day. I was not going to just play *at* tennis. I was going to *be* a tennis player.

From that day I never once struggled with my weight. Tennis became the first thing that went down on my daily schedule. I found I had plenty of time to do everything else once that had been scheduled. I had been kidding myself about "no time" all of my life. I was so excited about the process of being a tennis player that I never had a moment's doubt about my ultimate success and weight loss. I *knew* I would succeed. Sure, I dieted. But this time, I joked about dieting. I invented the Four-S Diet: unlimited indulgence in shrimp, steak, salad, and sex. The diet was something of an exaggeration, of course, since I just cut out desserts, cut way down on fats, and nibbled on fruit and vegetables whenever I felt hungry. I would restrict calories for maybe a month at a time. Then I would eat normally. My new level of activity prevented me from regaining any weight. Then I would cut back again on calories for another three or four weeks. It was simply no problem sticking to a diet for a few weeks and then maintaining my weight with an active lifestyle.

The key to my own success lies in the word *be*, when I speak of "being a tennis player." I was not playing *at* the game. *Being* a tennis player became a central part of my self-concept, just as being a runner today is also part of my self-concept. I don't do these things for weight control or for my health. Through them, I express previously hidden aspects of myself—strength and skills I never knew I had as a fat man.

There lies sleeping in even the most sedentary body a capacity for running, jumping, and playing that, once developed and expressed, satisfies some basic biological need and gives unparalleled pleasure. I do not believe anyone who has always been thin and fit can appreciate the contrast and experience physically and psychologically what the change to a thin and active life from a fat sedentary existence provides. And for fat people, an active fantasy and imagination can provide a sense of their future potential which sustains their motivation to change.

In spite of my own experience, however, I never appreciated the role of fantasy and the importance of having a goal in life that required a thin body until the day Cindy told me her story. Cindy struggled, as many of you may have to struggle. I didn't because of the pleasure I got from tennis. Dieting became rewarding because I would sense the improvement in my ability to move and in my endurance with every few pounds lost. And, as an additional aid during my dieting episodes, whenever anyone asked me why I was passing up alcohol, or desserts, I simply told them about my new Four-S Diet. That was good for a few laughs, and my hosts at dinner parties or my restaurant companions never urged me to eat anything I didn't want to after that.

The only problem I had to face, one that you may know as well as I, was my embarrassment over my body. I, too, thought I was ugly. For a full year, I wore long pants on the tennis court, even in

95° heat or hotter. I never changed clothes at the gym. I didn't want anyone to see the way I looked. But when I broke 200 pounds (I now weigh 154), I took a giant leap forward and bought my first pair of tennis shorts. The same day, I took my first shower at the gymnasium.

Yes, I have stretch marks and a little loose skin in the hip area. After all, I went from fifty-five inches around my hips to thirty-nine inches. (I have the hand-tailored pants made for me when I was twenty-three years old, still hanging in my closet to prove it.) But the rest of me tightened up, in part because I lost weight slowly and got active. Unless I exhibit my old clothes, no one can believe I was a fat man until I was thirty-five years old.

Now it's time for you, too, to get moving. Pull out those fantasies about living in a strong and active body. If you have ever secretly wished to be or look like a dancer or an athlete, just start spending forty-five minutes each day doing what they do, and your body will begin to shape itself in that mold. It will continue to shape itself to its full genetic potential.

I'll show you how to get started in the next two chapters. I can't promise that you will ever become a great dancer or an Olympic-class athlete, but you will in the end be able to eat pretty much to your heart's content.

5

THE GOOD MORNING ROUTINE

Flexibility and Strength

There are three components to physical fitness: flexibility, muscular strength, and cardiovascular endurance. Activities that increase cardiovascular endurance (walking, jogging, swimming, bicycling, continuous dancing, or play at racquet sports) are the ones that burn the most calories and elevate your metabolic rate. They are therefore essential to weight loss and maintenance.

In the rush to lose weight and increase cardiovascular health, many people overemphasize cardiovascular activities and slight the development of flexibility and strength. That is unfortunate for many reasons. Flexibility and strengthening exercises have their own unique cosmetic effects. They also make the lifting, carrying, and shoving tasks of daily living easier. Increased suppleness and strength reduce the likelihood of accidents such as slipping and falling, or throwing your back out. They also decrease the possibility of injury if you decide to increase the intensity or duration of your cardiovascular activities. And finally, developing flexibility and strength produce their own psychological benefits.

The beginning fitness program described in this chapter and the next is designed to get you into such good shape that you will come to enjoy activity and feel confident about your physical ability. You will have the courage and desire to try any number of games or physical activities until you do find one that stimulates you. The best physical activity for you is one that makes you feel good and that you can fantasize about. It may be one that fulfills a childhood dream.

Graduates of this basic program end up doing many things: aerobic dancing, swimming, tennis, walking, jogging, racquet ball, yoga, bicycling, even karate. As soon as you understand the basic principles and learn to trust your own body and personal inclinations you will design your own program. No two people, even after a few weeks, are doing quite the same stretches, the same body building exercises, or the same aerobic activities.

The program I describe in these two chapters is safe for anyone in good health and is likely to be exactly what your doctor will recommend in most cases even if you are not. It is all any adult needs to do to lose weight, keep it off, and become physically fit. However, if you have cardiac disease, hypertension, diabetes, arthritis, lower back pain, or joint injuries that can make movement painful, you should consult your physician. You may need some special preparatory or remedial exercise before building to the level I suggest. Persons with severe hypertension should be cautious about lifting weight and some stretches can aggravate chronic back pain. I'll show you what to look for as we go along and how to become strong and flexible without injury.

Use These Principles to Enhance
the Pleasure of Activity

Here are some principles that have helped getting fit and staying active become a pleasure for many overweight people who never thought exercise was anything but a pain or a bore. Try them out, but remember, we are each unique. Once you begin to trust your own feelings and judgment, you may want to do many things that are different from these recommendations. Fine. But if you have never enjoyed being active before, use these principles to guide your first efforts. They may make the difference.

1. *Pay attention to your bodily sensations.* Feel each stretch, notice how your body reacts to each movement. Focus on the way your muscles feel as you do the light weight work. Watch the difference each day. As you see what your body can do and how it changes, confidence in your physical powers will grow.

2. *Avoid competition—at least at the onset.* I admit that I take pride in the fact that some of my former weight group participants, even fifty- to sixty-year-olds, are distance racing and winning. Others

jog, or even walk in races, just for the companionship and exhilaration it brings. Can you imagine running a five- or ten-mile race? They couldn't either. My own pride is nothing compared to their satisfaction.

However, competition can hurt you physically and mentally. You may have tremendous hidden potential, but being overweight puts you at an initial disadvantage. Don't even *compare* yourself to anyone else, not in dance class, on the road, or on the tennis court. Start with the attitude that you are doing this for yourself and no one else. And wait to discover what signals your body sends you as you progress. Once you get in shape, you may indeed find that competition suits your temperament and keeps you looking forward to the next event. For now, just . . .

3. *Set your own personal standards.* I tell my patients at the beginning, *"Do, but underdo."* I mean by this to keep doing, but *never* try to hit maximum. Do just enough today to make you eager and fit to be active tomorrow. Do enough to give you the feeling that you are improving. Examine your progress in a long-time perspective—weeks, if not months. On those days when you seem to lack energy for whatever reason and don't seem to be quite as vigorous as the day before, remember that we have often to drop back a step or two before we can make a leap forward.

4. *Go by time.* Do not set quantity, speed, or distance goals at the start of this program. In the flexibility routine, mentally set aside the amount of time you are going to spend, then feel your way to find the most pleasurable tempo. Don't try to squeeze umpteen movements into a brief period to get them over with. Most of us rush enough the rest of the day; rushing is a sure way to make exercise distasteful.

5. *Try a meditational attitude as you flex and stretch.* By focusing on your bodily sensations, moving at your own special tempo, and gently excluding extraneous thoughts, you can finish a fifteen-minute session with the same refreshing mental benefits of a period of yogic meditation.

6. *Seek variety.* Some people lock into a routine and never deviate. It seems perfect for them. But most prefer some variety. Learn the Good Morning Routine first. Follow it religiously until it becomes second nature. It will develop the flexibility and strength that prepare you for other things. Then go to chapter thirteen and add

variety to your own program. Or, buy the books I suggest. Or, take
an honest-to-goodness yoga class. Or, join the Y. In several weeks—
let us say ten or twelve at the most—you will have developed the
strength, flexibility, cardiovascular endurance, and the *courage* to
do any of these things without embarrassment. You will also have
tested my principles, lost at least twenty pounds of fat, and be prepared to really *enjoy* formal classes or instruction of any kind.

7. *Talk to others about your program.* Talking about your commitment reinforces your resolve. You will find others who will want to
learn from you and others you can learn from. You may find some
new friends and exercise companions in this way.

WARNING: If you think you are going to have a scheduling
problem with activities, *do not start this activity program until you turn
to chapter seven and carry out a simple life management analysis.* You
might enjoy doing this analysis even if you already know how to
plan everything you want to accomplish and accomplish most of
what you plan. *Do not start this activity program unless you are ready to
commit yourself to it on a daily basis.* I'll help you keep renewing that
commitment. But if you are not ready to be active in one way or
another every day—if you are not 100 percent ready to give yourself a chance to see if you can benefit from what I have to offer—
then just give this book to someone else. Perhaps it can help them
and you will have done a good deed!

The Good Morning Routine

The Good Morning Routine combines flexibility and strength.
It is preceded by three warm-up exercises. I will describe each group
of exercises separately, and, as I go along, I will indicate their
rationale, along with other comments. Normally, people like to mix
up the order of these exercises. When you know them well, mix
them up in any way that pleases you.

Depending upon how long you hold each stretch, or how many
repetitions you do of a strengthening exercise, the routine takes
between ten and fifteen minutes. You can do these exercises at any
time during the day, but there is a special reason to do at least some
of them when you get up in the morning. During my description
of the exercises, I will explain why.

You can take a minute's rest between exercises whenever you feel like it. You can do some exercises in the bathroom, some in the kitchen, some in the dining area, completing them as you get ready for breakfast and prepare to go to work.

Warm-ups

These three exercises are best done more or less continuously, flowing one into the other. Pay attention to your body—it will tell you how many repetitions you need each day. This number may vary. I will make some suggestions.

1. **Arm Swings**   Swing your arms from side to side, rotating your upper body from the hips. Let your arms flap freely, so that when you turn to the left, your right hand slaps against your left shoulder and your left hand, crossing behind you, slaps against your right hip or lower back. When you turn left, look over your left shoulder; when you turn right, look over your right shoulder. Keep loose. A dozen swings to each side, give or take a few, will do it. You will know when to stop—you will begin to feel good in your lower back and spine.

2. **Reach for the Stars**   Bring both arms above your head. Keeping your right heel on the floor, stretch high with your right hand, and feel the pull from your right hip, along your right side, and into your right shoulder. This stretch improves if you can raise your left heel off the ground, slightly bending your left knee, as you stretch the right hand upward. Reverse sides, stretching left hand up, keeping left heel down, and raising right heel. If you get confused about your feet, forget it. Just stretch each arm up and pull out on each side as you do this. Six or so stretches on each side does it for most people. Nice and slow.

3. **Bendover**   Curl down, *keeping knees slightly bent* for this warm-up. Let your arms just dangle toward the floor. You do not need to touch the floor. This is a relaxed dangle. Some people wiggle a little at the hips to help let loose in the lower back and hip area. If you do this stretch in the morning, you are likely to be stiff, so do not force it. Hold twelve to twenty seconds. Curl up slowly, straightening one vertebra at a time.

Always remember to breathe naturally and normally as you exercise.

EX. 1 *Arm Swings*

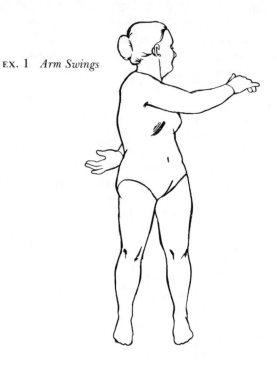

EX. 2 *Reach for the Stars*

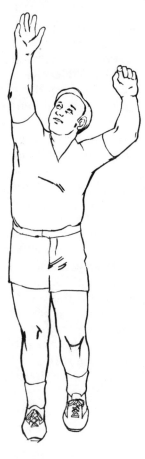

EX. 3 *Bendover*

The three warm-up stretches take about one minute—just about enough time to get hot water up from the water heater to the faucet if you do it in the bathroom.

I recommend you try the meditational framework for body movement. It will set you up for a calm, self-controlled day.

Concentrate your attention on your bodily feelings. If any thoughts intrude, just focus again on your bodily sensations and see what meaning they begin to assume for you. As your body awareness grows, these exercises will become especially valuable and satisfying.

The Stretching Sequence

In the following stretching exercises, go to the point where you begin to feel the stretch. Then, rest there, relaxing *into* the stretch. Yoga teachers use the expression "playing around the edge" of a stretch.

4. *Side Stretch*   With feet at shoulder width, raise right arm straight overhead, and bend sideways to the left. Feel the stretch, and stop there. Hold it for twelve to twenty seconds. Keep breathing normally. Then return to upright position and repeat to the right side. You may find with this exercise, as with others, that one side of the body is tighter than the other.

5. *Calf Stretch*   Stand arm's length from a wall. Move left leg a half step toward the wall, and the right leg a half step back. Keeping the right heel on the floor, lean forward and put hands against the wall, keeping the right leg straight. (The left knee is bent.) Feel the stretch in the right calf muscle. It helps the stretch to keep your back and rear end in line with the straight leg. If you do not feel any pull, inch your right leg back a ways, keeping the heel flat, until you do. Hold twelve to twenty seconds.

Now, still in approximately the same position, bend slightly at the waist, sticking your rump out to the rear. Then bend the right knee to flex the ankle and stretch the Achilles tendon. You should feel the stretch starting at the ankle and proceeding up the rear of the leg to the calf muscle. Keep your heel flat. Hold twelve to twenty seconds. Reverse your leg position and repeat with the left leg back and the right foot forward.

6. *Hamstring Stretch*   Lift right leg up and place it on a convenient surface—a chair, table top, or counter. It is perfectly fine to

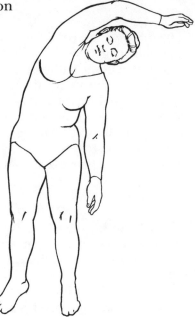

EX. 4   *Side Stretch*

EX. 5a   *Calf Stretch* (first position)   EX. 5b   *Calf Stretch* (second position)

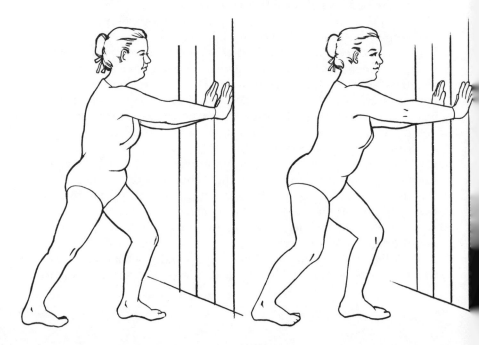

start with a low surface—even a footstool. As you lose weight it will feel good to get the leg up higher. Keep your back straight and head in line. Lean slowly forward until you feel a pull on the hamstring muscles along the under part of your thigh. Hold for twelve to twenty seconds. You can rest your arms on your knee, your foreleg, or hold on to your ankle as you lean. Some people reach their toes. Go far enough forward to feel a pull. Reverse legs.

7. *Back Extension and Forward Bend*   Place palms on the small of your back, bend knees slightly, and thrust your pelvis forward. Then lean backwards, dropping your head back and pushing upwards and backwards with your chin. You are trying to look back over your head. Arch only enough to feel the stretch in the lower back. Support yourself well with your hands. Hold for five to ten seconds to begin with.

Come up slowly and curl down in a forward bend. This time you can keep your knees straight if it feels good and if your back is loose. With straight legs you will feel the stretch in your lower back and in your hamstrings again. Hold as long as it feels good, perhaps five to ten seconds.

Do not be tempted (or pressured by anyone) to do a forward bend with legs perfectly straight, lunging to touch the floor, until you know that hamstrings and back are flexible enough to do it without pain. You may need to keep a slight flex in your knees for a couple of weeks. Your flexibility will increase gradually, and you can gradually straighten your knees. Let your fingers just touch your forelegs as low as they can comfortably. Gradually you will find your fingers touching nearer your ankles, then on the tops of your feet, then your toes, then the floor. Soon you will be ready to enjoy more advanced yogic stretching (chapter thirteen). (Do not do forward bends with straight legs if you have chronic lower back pain. See the sitting back stretch exercise in chapter thirteen for a substitute.)

8. *Quadriceps Stretch*   Holding on to a chair or counter top, bring your right knee up towards your chest until you can grab your ankle or your foot over the instep. Then, bring the foot back around towards your rear to the point where the right thigh is in line with the left leg. Try to touch your rear with your heel. You should feel the stretch in the front part of the thigh. To increase the stretch, you can extend the foot away from you, slightly arching

EX. 6 *Hamstring Stretch*

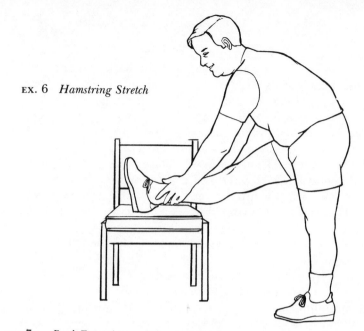

EX. 7a. *Back Extension and Forward Bend*
(first position)

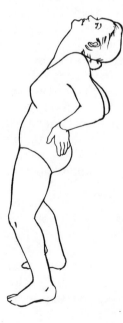

EX. 7b *Back Extension and Forward Bend*
(second position)

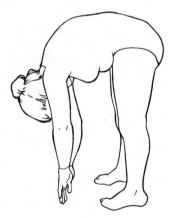

EX. 8 *Quadriceps Stretch*

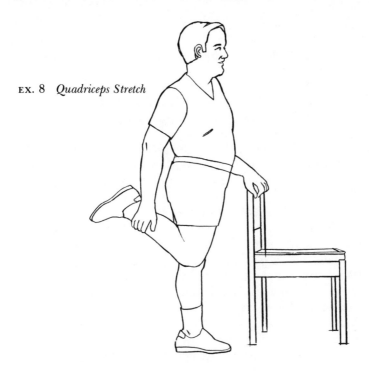

EX. 9 *Leg Raises, Foot Flexions, and Rotations*

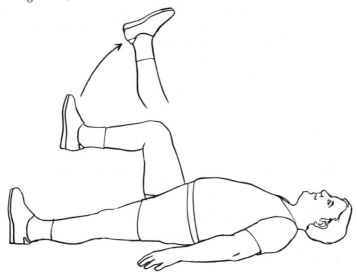

your back, and still holding the foot or ankle. Hold ten to twelve seconds and then reverse legs.

These next four exercises are done on the floor or in bed. They are *very, very* important for the beginning walker and jogger.

9. *Leg Raises, Foot Flexions, and Rotations*   Lying on the floor, raise your left leg from the hip joint until it is as close to being perpendicular to your body as is comfortable. Then, bending it at the knee, lower the foreleg until it is parallel to the floor. Raise your foreleg back up to the extended position and feel the contraction throughout the quadriceps, especially at the points that attach at the upper part of the knee joint. Hold for a second before bending back to parallel position. Repeat about ten times, or until you feel a slight strain. Return the foreleg to the bent position and flex the foot forward and backwards about ten times slowly. Then, rotate the foot at the ankle about six times in each direction. Lower the leg and repeat with the right leg. You are working here to prevent knee problems and shin splints.

10. *Partial Sit-up and Leg Lift*   This exercise can be done while you are still on the floor, right after or before the leg raise exercise above. Start with arms overhead and legs straight forward lying flat on the floor. Bring both knees to your chest (feet off the floor) and at the same time bring your arms forward. Raise only your head and shoulders from the floor. Hold a couple of seconds or until you feel the strain in your stomach area. Then place your feet on the floor and slide them forward, touching the floor as they go. Simultaneously, lower your head and shoulders and bring your arms back over your head. Repeat several times, or until you feel your stomach has done its share of the day's work.

This exercise is a substitute for sit-ups, which many overweight people cannot do, and most hate to do even if they can. Fortunately, it accomplishes all the things that sit-ups can do: it flattens the stomach as it increases the strength of the abdominal muscles and helps prevent lower back pain. It is even better for you than sit-ups because it uses the entire range of stomach muscles, and you can control your muscular exertion more easily. It also will not injure your tailbone, as sit-ups sometimes do.

When the version above becomes too easy, you can increase the effort by lessening your foot contact with the floor as you return to the extended position. In time, you may be able to do the exercise

EX. 10a *Partial Sit-up and Leg Lift*
(first position)

EX. 10b *Partial Sit-up and Leg Lift*
(second position)

EX. 10c *Partial Sit-up and Leg Lift*
(third position)

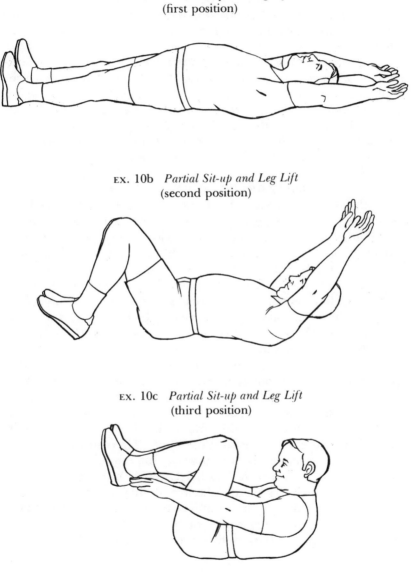

without allowing your feet or your head to touch the floor at all in the extended position. You hold yourself a few seconds in the extended position as well as in the curled position. A half dozen repetitions of this exercise can be as valuable as fifty sit-ups. The fact that it will take inches off your waist is quite incidental to the value it has in increasing abdominal strength and preventing back troubles.

This exercise, like many others that help prevent injury and pain, *can also aggravate existing troubles.* This is an unfortunate truth applicable to all fitness conditioning. *A normal stretching or strengthening exercise is often not applicable, at first, as a remedial exercise.* If you have back trouble, use the exercise prescribed by your physician or physical therapist until you are healed. Then you can proceed to higher levels of fitness with the standard exercises.

Shaping and Strengthening Sequence

With respect to strength, the upper body is frequently the most neglected part of our anatomy. Compared with the requirements of life just two or three generations back, few tasks today require much lifting, carrying, and pushing. If you find yourself getting tired carrying a few sacks of groceries, a suitcase, or even your child around, it only goes to prove my point. You are not in condition; you do not have enough reserve strength to make these tasks feel easy. And how can you expect to have firm looking arms and a firm bustline, if you never do anything that makes for strong, toned muscles in the arms, shoulders, and chest?

If you have neglected your arms, chest, and back muscles, the initial effects of the following exercises are quick and quite dramatic, especially mentally. When I ask people who have begun a strength training program, even one or two weeks later, how they feel, their reaction is universally the same. They bring their hands up and cross them in front of their chest. Then spreading them outward in a sweeping motion, they say something like, "I feel *so* much stronger and broader up here." Their posture changes as they speak. Their backs straighten and they stand taller, with shoulders squared. It is almost impossible not to like yourself better. These internal changes precede by several weeks any obvious contour changes, but they motivate you to continue your new routine.

In order to perform these exercises, you will need a couple of books. As soon as you know that you will never stop doing them, if you are a woman, you may prefer to use a five-pound or three-kilo (6.6 pound) set of dumbbells. Men prefer to use five-kilo (11 pound) weights. Dumbbells can be obtained cheaply from your local sporting goods store or a discount house. They tend to cost around ten dollars. Outside of a good pair of walking shoes, this is all the equipment you will need for this program.

Here is what the strength training exercises, and those in chapter thirteen accomplish:

By using a fairly large number of repetitions with light weight, you tone your muscles. That is, you increase their aliveness. They learn to react easily and quickly. You delineate their lines *without* increasing bulk.* And in addition to good-looking lines and increased responsivity of the muscle, you get significantly stronger as well.

When you first begin to use a muscle, central nervous system impulses are capable of recruiting only a limited portion of the muscle fibers in a given muscle group. By repeating the command, that is through practice, more and more of the existing fibers in the muscle begin to respond with each lift. Soon you can lift greater amounts or repeat a motion more times without fatigue. The total mass of the muscle increases, too, but it does not take on a bulky appearance.

It is a standard principle in weight lifting: long, well-delineated lines come from doing more repetitions with a light weight. Bulk develops from using such heavy weights that eight to twelve repetitions will bring you to the point of absolute exhaustion. Most people do not find this bulk attractive and get little enjoyment from this kind of lifting. In addition, working to exhaustion with a heavy weight is not generally safe for many adults. It causes a sharp increase in blood pressure. Only well-conditioned people in excellent health should work with heavy weights. Everyone can use the light weights I suggest and significantly improve their condition.

If you use books as weights for these exercises, pick two matched volumes of any comfortable weight, perhaps about three pounds.

* Bulk is increased significantly only through very heavy weight lifting and then only in men. An increase in bulk requires a high level of testosterone, the hormone that stimulates muscle growth. Only men have high levels of this hormone.

Hold the books *extended* away from your hands (*not* inside the palm facing up along the wrist and arm). Books do not need to be as heavy as dumbbells because, by extending them out from your hands, the effective load on the muscles is greater.

11. *The Shoulder Threesome* Hold weights at your side, with palms facing toward the rear. Keeping arms straight, raise weights forward to shoulder height and return to down position, slowly and with control. Repeat until you feel a moderate strain in the shoulder area. If you feel no effort, you have not gone on long enough; if you hurt, you have gone too far. For these and all strength-training exercises, a moderate pace is best. *Always breathe normally.* After you complete the forward series, rest one deep breath with arms at side, then, turn the weight so that the palms face your body. Raise outward to the side, to shoulder level. Return to down position. These exercises are harder. Continue repetitions until the point of moderate strain. Rest one deep breath. Then, bend forward at your waist until your upper body is parallel to the ground. Face palms toward each other with the weights hanging down in front of you. Raise weights to the side, to shoulder height, and return. These exercises are somewhat easier than the upright sideward motion. Rest at least one or two deep breaths and go on to the next exercise.

12. *Biceps Curl* Stand straight with arms at side, palms facing forward. Raise weights by curling forearms up to the shoulder. Return. Repeat at controlled and moderate pace until you feel some effort. Always add just one more repetition after the effort becomes noticeable, but do not strain to a maximum effort. By adding just one more repetition whenever the spirit moves you, you will significantly increase your strength without hurting yourself and without bringing on muscle soreness.

13. *Triceps* Bending from your hips, go forward to about a sixty-degree angle from the upright position. Bring elbows next to your body. Keeping upper arms parallel to and close to your trunk, bring weights to the shoulders with palms facing each other. Straighten forearms down and back behind your body, keeping upper arms still and always parallel and tucked next to your trunk. Bring forearms forward and up to the shoulders. This builds the triceps, that muscle at the rear of your upper arm, and will help reduce the

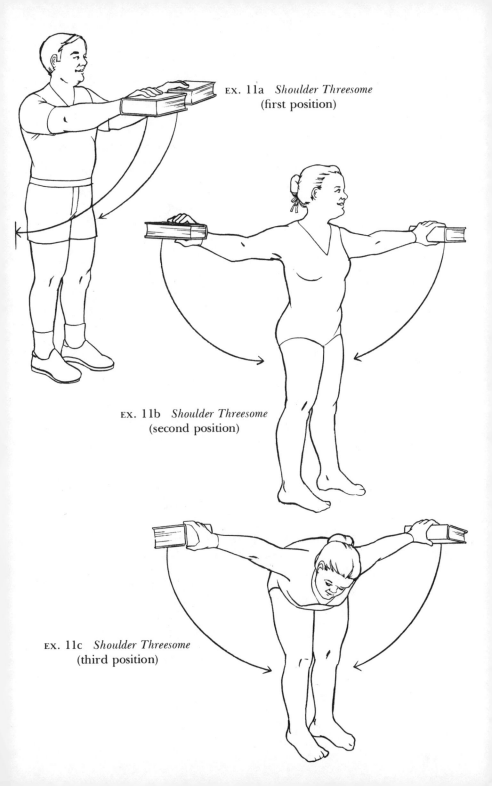

EX. 11a *Shoulder Threesome*
(first position)

EX. 11b *Shoulder Threesome*
(second position)

EX. 11c *Shoulder Threesome*
(third position)

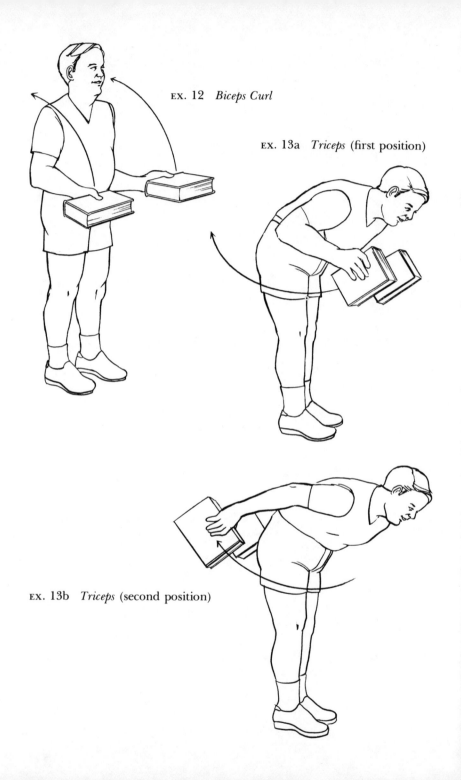

EX. 12 *Biceps Curl*

EX. 13a *Triceps* (first position)

EX. 13b *Triceps* (second position)

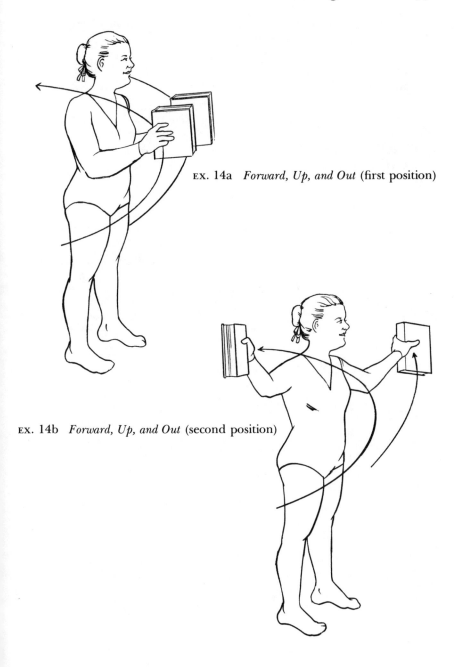

EX. 14a *Forward, Up, and Out* (first position)

EX. 14b *Forward, Up, and Out* (second position)

likelihood of loose-hanging skin on your upper arms as you lose body fat. Repeat until you feel moderate strain.

14. *Forward, Up, and Out*   Return to the upright standing position. Start with arms at sides, palms facing body. Curling at the elbows, bring weights forward and up almost to the shoulder level. Continue in one uninterrupted motion, spreading arms out to your side. At this point, your palms are facing forward. Keep your elbows slightly bent, even at the fullest extension. Return weights to the body at shoulder height and lower to your side. Repeat until slight strain is felt.

FOR THE LEGS

15. *Heel Lifts*   With weights at side (or for variety, held up at shoulder height, next to your body) go up and down slowly on your toes several times. Rest about a second at the top of the rise. The exercise helps shape calves. This is even better done with balls of

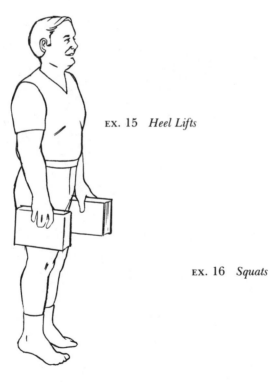

EX. 15   *Heel Lifts*

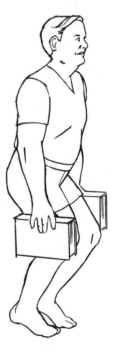

EX. 16   *Squats*

the feet up on a book or piece of two-by-four wood. You get more extension at the heel.

16. *Squats*   If you are significantly overweight (more than thirty pounds), you don't need extra weights for this exercise at first and it is better not to use them. As soon as you know that your knees will not hurt (and if you do this as I suggest, they are not likely to) you can add weight. In the end, adding weight is what contributes to your strength reserve. With arms at sides, feet at shoulder width, toes facing slightly out, squat down one-third to one-half of the way. *Do not go beyond the point where your thighs are parallel to the floor.* Heels can remain on the floor or can come up a bit—whatever feels right—as you go down. Return to the standing position. Repeat several times or until you feel some strain. This exercise can be done profitably with your heels up on a book or a two by four. If your knees hurt, do not do this exercise. Replace it with extra leg raises in the reclining position (number nine).

For the first week or two be sure to hold yourself back. Do all of these exercises gently and repeat only a few times. This will prepare your body to begin to build without any particular soreness and without injury. Resist the temptation to go fast or to see how many repetitions you can do for a particular exercise. That behavior courts disaster, physically and mentally. Within two weeks your flexibility will have increased. So will your circulation to those parts of the body that you may be using this way for the first time in many years. Then you can begin to think about increasing the repetitions of the muscular endurance exercises and the length or intensity of your stretches. Then you will discover the good feelings that fitness buffs rave about.

If you note any particular persistent pain—especially in your joints or lower back—check with your doctor because you may need some special advice. Don't stop, however, because of slight soreness. That will disappear and it will not recur when you begin gradually to increase your routine.

The Enemies Within

If you are like most overweight people, you must learn to deal with two enemies that exist side-by-side within you as you try to change: lethargy and impatience. Lethargy is the enemy that has kept you fat. But impatience lurks in the background, waiting to attack you when you try to overcome lethargy. How many times in the past, in your desire for overnight success, have you been overwhelmed by your impatience? Now, in your desire to be strong and fit before the body's due time, impatience can defeat you once again. Remember that the longest journey begins with one step. Take one step each day, *but never fail to take that step*. This is your assurance that you will complete the journey. But two quick steps, and impatience will defeat you once again. You will overdo and hurt yourself, or you will fail to discover that particular psychological benefit that comes from the slow, more reflective approach to fitness and body awareness that I urge you to pursue. With patience, you may discover that this approach is particularly suited to your temperament. It is certainly the best way to begin.

The Best Time for These Exercises

Any time, of course.

But, there is a unique benefit to the morning. Even if you do not do the whole series, there is a special, almost magical, psychological advantage to doing something different from your past routine immediately upon arising. A change in your behavior first thing in the morning demonstrates that you have made a commitment to change your life.

Beginning the day with some new ritual has another psychological benefit. Recall for a moment some of the rituals of your childhood. For example, walking on the sidewalk, attempting either to miss all the cracks or to hit every one of them, or throwing a pebble at a tree. Good things were going to happen to you if you were able to carry out your intentions. Even if you missed the first time, you went back and did it again to make sure you succeeded. Then you went about your business feeling good about yourself. You may have had some other game with an intent similar to this. But whatever, starting tomorrow, by doing something different immediately upon arising, even if it is only the three warm-ups—one teensy-weensy little minute—you can set the stage for changing your life. True, the entire act is yet to follow, but you can go about behaving the rest of the day with hope and determination.

This small change in your behavior becomes a symbol, an

expression of your commitment and firm resolution. It is the *first* expression of your intent to change *all* of those behaviors that have made you fat and kept you fat. It is the first step toward eating wisely and carrying out the rest of your activity plan. It is your secret weapon, an amulet, or magic wand.

It works because this one simple little act shows that you have *power*. You can change. Even if you are late for work or harassed by any household responsibility, you *do* have time for a few arm swings, a stretch, and a bend. If necessary, the rest of the routine can come later. As you do the three warm-ups in the bathroom or kitchen, you illustrate that you have the strength to control your body and that you are ready to sally forth and do battle with the temptations around you and the enemies within for the rest of the day.

So, beginning tomorrow, take this one step that you can take each day toward the building of a new you and a new life as a thinner, fitter individual. And as the day goes on, whenever you need to, you can recall the fact that you carried out this intention.

This is what willpower is made of. It is a series of little steps, small changes in your behavior, attached to a positive thought or self-evaluative statement. If you can force yourself to do something different when you get up tomorrow morning, how can you say that you don't have willpower?

You may think that other victories will be harder to achieve. You will find that you are wrong if you employ the strategies I suggest. Many changes must be brought about gradually. You simply select some small segment of your behavior, something that may take only a minute to begin with, and change it. To become a concert violinist, or pianist, the student must practice tiny motions in the same exercises and musical selections every day for many years until he or she achieves the required proficiency. Everyone accepts that fact. But when we want to lose weight and get fit, we want to have it happen as of yesterday. Just as physical skills and strength are built through the practice of certain daily tasks, so is willpower. It is a discipline, of course, but there is not a soul in the world who could not have a will of steel if he went about it one step at a time. Each step demonstrates your willpower and each step makes you slimmer and physically more fit.

So, let's begin. You are about to discover that activity changes are *far* more significant in helping you reach your goal than eating changes.

Here are two different sequences for the Good Morning Routine with which to experiment. Except for the warm ups, you can mix them up in any way that pleases you. You can always do numbers nine and ten in bed.

I	II
1.–3. Warm-ups	1.–3. Warm-ups
4. Side Stretch	4. Side Stretch
7. Back Extension	7. Back Extension
9. Leg Raises, Foot Flexions, Rotations	11. Shoulder Threesome
10. Partial Sit-ups and Leg Lifts	15. Heel Lifts
15. Heel Lifts	12. Biceps Curl
16. Squats	16. Squats
5. Calf Stretch	13. Triceps
6. Hamstring Stretch	14. Forward, Up, and Out
8. Quadriceps Stretch	9. Leg Raises, Foot Flexions, Rotations
11. Shoulder Threesome	10. Partial Sit-ups and Leg Lifts
12. Biceps Curl	8. Quadriceps Stretch
13. Triceps	5. Calf Stretch
14. Forward, Up, and Out	6. Hamstring Stretch

BURNING CALORIES: LEAVING FAT IN YOUR FOOTSTEPS

"I cannot imagine anyone walking or jogging four or five miles at a time. Isn't it boring? And besides, I could never run that far."

"Jogging is an essential part of my life. I actually have to force myself to take a day off each week. On that day I take a walk!"

These statements were made by the same person, the second some eighteen months later and twenty-two pounds lighter. Similar statements are being repeated daily all over this country by men and women who have discovered the almost mystical pleasure that accompanies walking and jogging. You, too, can discover a pleasurable route to weight control as well as excellent physical condition.

Here is the formula that can produce similar dramatic changes in your attitudes and feelings. Whether you end up as a committed walker or a confirmed jogger some time down the road, the formula is the same.

On the physical side, the body needs to build a capacity for

1. Forty to sixty minutes of steady state aerobic activity
2. Done at 60 to 70 percent of your maximum heart rate
3. With occasional periods of greater intensity activity done at whim, but never long enough or hard enough to cause injury.

On the mental side, the mind needs

1. To make a commitment to a plan of action strong enough to get through a probationary period that may last six months or a year

2. To start replacing food and dieting thoughts with information and ideas relevant to an active lifestyle

3. To learn to let loose, spin free, and fantasize.

How to Start

If you are like most people, you do not care to learn a lot of technical facts and jargon about physical activity.

Fortunately, walking is the simplest and most convenient way to implement my formula for what the mind and body need. And, fortunately, walking for enjoyment and for those valuable incidental byproducts, weight control and fitness, requires no rules. All you need to learn is to trust the signals your body sends you. Just get out and walk, searching for a style and a pace, and the attractive routes, that make you feel good.

Although walking for pleasure requires no rules, there is some information that may prove interesting and helpful. It is only natural to seek some guidance when you begin something new, and after all, I have a stake in seeing that you are successful.

It is worth remembering, however, that the great walkers of the past, from Socrates, Plato, and Aristotle, through Emerson, Thoreau, and Wordsworth, to Russell and Einstein of more recent times, knew nothing about exercise physiology, training heart rates, and the like. I am not sure it would have mattered to them either. They did it by "feel," and they all considered their daily walks to be an essential ingredient of their lives, the foundation of their health and their mental productivity.

The physical and psychological requirements that I have enumerated in the formula are implemented simultaneously and interact to bring you to your desired goal. Here is how to go about it.

What the Body Needs

Endurance

You need to build a capacity for forty to sixty minutes of activity because it is someplace within this period of time that a great majority of people experience the psychological and physical benefits of activity.

Some people feel great after about forty minutes; others cannot force themselves to stop much short of an hour once they discover the rewards of walking (or jogging, swimming, and bicycling). You will discover your personal range as you build your capacity. Preferred times for things like dancing and racquet sports also require similar physical capacity, but depend as well on social and skill factors for enjoyment.

I want to concentrate on walking as my example because I consider walking to be about the best activity for weight loss and the best for getting yourself into shape to do other things later on, if you choose.

In order to get to forty minutes, or more of walking, you must begin gradually. If you are significantly overweight, fifty pounds or more, test yourself with five minutes at a comfortable pace. Do it for two or three days. Then, if you have not experienced any ill effects, go for ten minutes, and continue at that level for a few days. Most people less than fifty pounds overweight can start with a fifteen-minute walk. Go at a steady, comfortable pace. Any time of the day is fine, but remember, to reach a goal of forty minutes or more takes time. Try fifteen-minute walks for two weeks, increase gradually to 30 minutes over the next two weeks, and go to forty-five minutes during the next two weeks. Listen to your body and trust the signals it sends you.

Why forty to sixty minutes? Do I need to do it all at once? How about two twenty-minute periods? How about a lot of short extra walking, such as parking farther from work and farther from the grocery store?

All of these things will burn calories and improve your health. Breaking it up is fine, and you should always walk as much as you can in performing your daily tasks anyway.

But a long walk has singular benefits. It permits the mind to clear. It allows the body to settle into a rhythm. It sets the stage for those changes in body chemistry that lead to some especially good feelings. Steady state aerobic activity seems to increase the production of endorphins, those internally produced morphinelike substances that directly affect mood. A steady state activity such as walking also appears to change the level of chemical nerve transmitting substances that may be related to stress and anxiety reduction.

After about forty-five minutes of aerobic activity, the state you have achieved lingers with you for as much as several hours. Perhaps that is why walkers and joggers seem so imperturbable—it is hard to rile anyone who feels so good.

About forty-five minutes of this activity appears to be an important preparation for the mental state called "spinning free" by Dr. Glasser. While one can pursue a direct line of thought and get a lot of work done while walking or jogging with this low level of effort, the steady rhythm of a walk gradually frees the mind to rove, as well as the feet. Creative solutions to problems appear. Bits of pleasant memories float by. Feelings for and about your body begin to change. For most people it takes at least twenty minutes to establish the flow, sometimes thirty, and then you need to stay there a while to savor it.

You will know you have reached the stage I am speaking of when it gets hard to stop once you've started. You will be sure you have reached it when the high point of your week is that special long walk with which you reward yourself on weekends.

Another benefit that follows from forty-five minutes of low intensity steady state aerobic activity is an increased ability to relax. Muscles that have exerted themselves react afterwards with more profound relaxation than can be obtained from almost any other means. Perhaps that is why one Zen master has said that meditation in motion is superior to meditation in repose. If you have become accustomed to using muscle relaxants and sleeping pills, there is an excellent chance you will throw them away as you go out for a walk sometime in the near future.

Finally, forty-five minutes or so of activity done almost every day, especially for walkers (joggers may do well taking one or two days a week off and varying their activities) seems to be essential to the "addiction process."

After a time, the daily walk becomes so much a part of the body's diurnal requirements—even more so than a particular pattern of eating—that to miss a day causes a yearning in our bones. Our body rhythms grow to depend upon our walk, just as they can become dependent on the more negative addictions such as smoking, and drinking alcohol or coffee.

I have been using the words "aerobic activity." By this we mean activity done in the presence of oxygen.* By steady state, we mean

---

*Activities such as weight lifting or sprinting at top speed use stored energy anaerobically—without oxygen. Energy that can be used this way is exhausted in a minute or two. Before you can repeat the movement, the quick energy supply must

a constant rate of oxygen consumption. Steady walking and gentle jogging are the two best ways for most people to enter into a steady state of moderate aerobic exertion. Although swimming is easier on the joints than walking or jogging, few people become proficient enough to do it at a steady, controlled intensity. Swimming is also a less convenient activity. Bicycling is excellent and a highly pleasurable activity, but outdoor cycling is sometimes dangerous, more at the mercy of the weather, and often not possible to do at a steady rate. Indoor cycling, on a stationary bicycle, is a good fallback activity in extremely bad weather. However, most people do not enjoy stationary bicycling as the mainstay of their cardiovascular fitness program.

Here is how moderate steady state aerobic activity affects caloric expenditure. Most people expend energy, burning glucose and fat, at a rate between 1 and 1.5 calories per minute just sitting still. This requires 200 to 300 milliliters of oxygen and is called your resting metabolic rate. When you walk steadily at three miles per hour, which is fast enough to be the basic speed at the start of any conditioning program, you burn approximately three times as many calories as you do sitting still—from 3 to 4.5 calories per minute. It requires three times as much oxygen. Thus, as long as you keep walking at that rate, you are performing a steady state aerobic activity that burns three times as many calories and requires three times as much oxygen as is consumed in your resting state.

The heart naturally has to work a bit harder to get this much oxygen around your system. So, it beats faster. In some people it goes up from a resting rate of 48 beats per minute to 54. In others, it goes up from a resting rate of 84 beats per minute to 138. In both cases, the heart and vascular systems are providing oxygen to

---

be replaced. You are considered to have an "oxygen debt" during this period, because oxygen is being used in large amounts to replenish that quick energy store from your long-term energy stores, even though your body is at rest. You are aware of being in oxygen debt because you continue to breathe hard after the exertion while this is going on.

All body movement has both aerobic and anaerobic components, but anything that can be sustained for long periods is primarily aerobic, while anything that exhausts you in just a few minutes is primarily anaerobic. When you first take up jogging, and you are out of condition, the movement is anaerobic because it exhausts you in a short time. But your aerobic powers improve; activities that first required anaerobic energy stores can be done aerobically. That is why training makes it possible to go faster for longer periods of time, up until your full potential for developing aerobic capacity is reached.

the body at about three times the resting rate. Why the tremendous difference in cardiovascular response? You probably guessed it. One person is lean and fit; the other fat and sedentary. The first person is hardly aware of any effort, but that second heart is having a relatively tough time. Fortunately, it can change.

Which brings me to the next point.

Aerobic Capacity

When a person begins to walk, moving out at a comfortable, moderate pace, breathing a little more deeply and a bit more quickly, but still easily able to carry on a conversation, the heart rate goes up just the right amount!

All those good things that accompany an increase in cardiovascular endurance begin to happen to the mind and to the body.

When you are walking for pleasure and for weight management, this is all you really need to know about such things as training heart rates and cardiovascular fitness.

But if you are interested in the technical particulars of cardiovascular training, *the best exercise heart rate at the beginning of a fitness program is 60 to 70 percent of your maximum possible heart rate.*

In general, a person's maximum heart rate lies close to a figure determined by subtracting your age from the number 220. Thus, most 30-year-olds have a maximum heart rate in the vicinity of 190; 50-year-olds around 170; etc.

These theoretical figures have been determined by exercising people of various ages at maximum exertion. At that point, the heart simply cannot go faster. The maximum attainable heart rate slows with age, as do many other bodily functions including basal metabolism. Having a maximum heart rate above or below the average for an age group does not seem to matter very much in terms of health or physical capacity for work.

Because few of us are in shape to go all out for a few minutes to determine our actual maximum heart rates, it is customary to use the theoretical figure obtained from research. It is a good working approximation.

The beneficial exercise heart rate range for beginners is determined by multiplying your maximum (220 minus your age) by .6 to obtain a lower level, and by .7 to obtain the upper level. Table 1 presents suggested heart rates by five-year age groups. These are called the training or target heart rates by fitness educators.

TABLE 1
Maximum Heart Rates and Target Zones

AGE	MAX. H.R. (BPM)	60% LEVEL (BPM)	70% LEVEL (BPM)	90% LEVEL (BPM)
20	200	120	140	180
25	195	117	137	176
30	190	114	133	171
35	185	111	130	167
40	180	108	126	162
45	175	105	123	158
50	170	102	119	153
55	165	99	116	149
60	160	96	112	144
65	155	93	108	140

Determine your approximate range by looking at the table. If you learn to take your pulse, I think you will find that what I have recommended will be your most enjoyable "cruising range" for walking. It is not too intense even for cardiac patients. And this walking speed is unlikely to be so fast that any orthopedic problems will arise unless you are more than fifty pounds overweight or have an existing problem. About three-miles-per-hour seems to do it for beginning walkers less than fifty pounds overweight. If you are heavier, it is imperative that you walk as slowly as is necessary to avoid such things as shin splints (inflammation that causes pain in your forelegs), back pain, and joint problems. And you *must* do your flexibility and muscle strengthening routines.

One convenient place to take your pulse is at the radial artery which lies on the inside of the wrist along a line to your thumb. Use two fingers of the other hand, usually the middle two, with light pressure. Do not use the other thumb because it may have its own pulse and confuse the count.

Count the beats for ten seconds and multiply by six to get your beats per minute (BPM).

Some people prefer to use the carotid artery, which can be felt in the neck in an indentation just to the side of the Adam's apple. Use two middle fingers.

Practice at rest a few times and note your resting heart rate. As you become active, that rate will tend to slow down. This occurs because the heart becomes capable of delivering a larger amount of blood with each beat (a larger stroke volume), and because the oxygen-carrying capacity of the blood improves. So does your muscle system's ability to use oxygen more efficiently. Ten and twenty percent reductions in resting heart rates are common, even more in a person who is seriously overweight and out of condition.

A few people may not show much of a reduction in resting heart rate. If you happen to be such a person it is nothing to be concerned about. *However, after two or three months of increased activity, virtually all people will show a reduction in their heart rates during the actual act of walking.*

You might find it interesting to monitor your own pulse while walking to watch your progress over these next ten or twelve weeks. I use an easy three-mile-per-hour walk test to monitor my patients. We simply go out from my office and walk around the block taking the pulse after about five or ten minutes. In the example I gave earlier, the woman who began the program with the pulse of 138 while walking during week one had reduced it to 114 by week twelve. *She was still expending three times the calories relative to her resting rate as she did three months earlier, walking at a similar rate of speed. But now her heart was working with almost 20 percent more efficiency.*

It may already have occurred to you that as your cardiovascular endurance increases, you are going to have to move a bit faster to get your heart rate up into that 60 to 70 percent cruising exercise range! Indeed, that is true. How much faster depends in part upon the biologically given limits to your cardiovascular capacity, how much activity you have been doing, and how much weight you lose. But, after a certain time, you will be finding it easier to move and to increase your pace. Then, at some new faster pace, you will experience no increased effort in your breathing and body as a whole. Upon taking your pulse, you will find that your heart is beating no faster at a three and a half or four mile-per-hour pace than it did at three miles-per-hour a few months before. To determine your degree of improvement you will have to force yourself to slow down to three miles-per-hour to take your pulse and compare it with your earlier records.

Most women take about twenty or twenty-one steps every ten seconds in order to walk at a three mile-per-hour clip. This increases to about twenty-seven or twenty-eight steps in ten seconds at four miles-per-hour. Men generally have a longer stride and take about sixteen or seventeen steps each ten seconds to reach three miles-per-hour, and twenty to twenty-one at four miles-per-hour.

If you are curious enough to be more scientific about your pace, try it out over a measured distance, or on a quarter-mile track. See how long it takes at your preferred speeds. It is amazing how quickly we learn to identify our preferred paces. Soon you will never need to clock yourself again to know how fast you are going. Without a watch, I have walked a mile at what my bones said was a three-mile-per-hour pace, and missed, according to my friend's chronograph, by only five seconds. On two other occasions which I doubt I could ever replicate so closely again, I have jogged what my body said were eight-minute- and eight-and-one-half-minute miles. I missed (very much to my surprise) by less than two seconds each time. I know several walkers and runners who hum different tunes to help set their paces. The tempo of each song is so well known that their pace will always be within a few seconds per mile each time they use their different tunes.

As you read other fitness books you will find that exercise physiologists and fitness experts tend to recommend higher workout ranges than I do. They typically suggest 70 to 85 percent, or even 90 percent of your maximum heart rate. For high level conditioning this may be necessary. You will be tempted to go faster too. It is unavoidable because speed has its own particular rewards. As you get thinner and more fit, you will not be able to repress your spirit. I have never met a person who could.

But I have also discovered that even the most committed long-distance walkers and joggers, those who enjoy the *process* of walking and running, do *most* of their activity in the 60 to 70 percent range. Only a part of their day's run is done at higher intensity. And only once or twice a week do they go anywhere near a 90 percent effort for any length of time. The 60 to 70 percent level appears to be the range in which good feelings *during* activity develop. The more intense effort, sometimes experienced as agony by competitive runners in training and while racing, pays off in exhilaration *after* it is over.

How do both conditioned runners and walkers end up in the same 60 to 70 percent of maximum heart rate range during exercise, yet move at such different speeds? Through training, the runners build greater cardiovascular capacity and endurance. A runner capable of an eight-miles-per-hour pace (a seven-and-a-half-minute mile) may cruise at a six-mile-per-hour pace (ten-minute mile) with a pulse of 102. A walker capable of five miles-per-hour (twelve minute mile) will cruise at four miles-per-hour (fifteen minute mile) with a similar rate of 102. Both enjoy their movements equally.

Just because runners can go faster does not mean that runners are healthier than walkers. It does not mean that runners have greater protection from cardiovascular disease or any other disease. It does not mean that runners are going to live longer. It only means that runners have trained their systems to go faster—that is all. And unless the runners have used good judgment they have increased the likelihood of injury far above that of walkers. Over 60 percent of runners injure themselves. Only a tiny fraction of walkers ever do. *In the long run, walkers may be healthier than runners.*

Nevertheless, the urge to go faster hits us all. An occasional greater load on our system will build our strength and frequently contributes to our enjoyment.

Picking up the Pace

I have suggested that you begin with any pace that feels good, which for most people is usually about a three mile-per-hour pace. (It will be even slower for very heavy people.) When you reach the point that you can continue for about forty-five minutes at this pace without ill effects and have done so for a week or two, it may be time to try to follow that irrepressible urge to add a little speed. However, there is certainly no need to go faster for the sake of fitness if your heart rate during walking at three miles per hour remains in that 60 to 70 percent of maximum range. That pace is all you need for your health, to add to your pleasure in living, and to manage your weight.

But I know the urge will surface and that giving in will be very gratifying. And done wisely, faster walking will increase your cardiovascular endurance and the strength of your legs. It also burns more calories. When you hit four miles per hour, you burn four-and-one-half to five times the calories you use sitting still.

Do not give in to the urge to move faster until you have a solid capacity for the three miles-per-hour speed. Then, pick up your pace for a brief period during your next walk—just a few minutes—and see how it feels. If you have carefully followed my advice to get your walking time up to forty-five minutes or so at three miles per hour before you pick up speed, your body will react with a rush of excitement. Instead of tiring quickly, you will respond to the speed with increased vigor.

But don't get carried away. Slow down and see if everything still feels fine. Let your breathing and heart settle back to their usual rates at the three mile-per-hour pace. Check your legs and see how your knees and ankles are doing. See how your calf and thigh muscles feel. If all systems continue to say "go," pick up speed again—but only for a few minutes. Then return to your base speed.

Begin to do this more frequently and for longer periods as the weeks progress. The physical reactions at your higher speed should still be pleasant—breathing becomes deeper and a little faster. There is never any need to get out of breath. Your main concern is never to exert to the point of joint pain, although after a long or faster walk some stiffness is to be expected. Just remember to use the flexibility routine I described in chapter five. Seriously overweight people must pay special attention to flexibility and strength to avoid injury and to build their capacities for walking.

If you take your pulse during your fast walking periods, it may go up into that 70 to 90 percent range suggested by most fitness experts. By now your body will be ready for it. When you begin to exercise at the higher intensity reflected in heart rates at 70 percent of maximum or above, conditioning proceeds faster and reaches higher levels, if that is what you want. But good health does not require it and orthopedic injuries become more likely. If you reach the point where you wish to break into a run, be sure to follow my advice on how to jog injury free (chapter thirteen).

Whether you end up a walker or a jogger is a matter of personal choice. That choice can be influenced by anatomical as well as psychological factors, as I know from personal experience.

One of my colleagues, Dr. John Pleas, is a confirmed walker. In training, he alternates hard days (eighteen miles) with light days (eight miles). He walked forty-one miles in twenty-four hours to celebrate his forty-first birthday last year and over seventy-five this year to celebrate his forty-second. Walking is a part of his life, just as jogging, tennis, and bicycling are more a part of mine. I, like the person I quoted at the start of this chapter, reserve a five-mile walk for my day off each week, and I definitely do enjoy the contrast with my other activities. But, in spite of my good overall condition, I cannot walk with John. His cruising pace for miles on end is over four miles per hour. The last time I went on a three-mile walk with him, I returned with pain in my lower back and right hip socket. The same thing happened to another jogger colleague of mine who tried to walk at John's pace. For some reason, it is easier for me to jog ten miles at a nine- or ten-minute-per-mile pace than it is to walk ten miles using any combination of paces. I have tried both. I am either not in condition for such walking, or I am not built as well for it as I am for jogging. I'll show you how to find out which will suit you best in chapter thirteen.

What the Mind Needs

Commitment

If you have read this far, you are probably on the verge of making a commitment to change something in order to lose weight and get fit. But you are no doubt wondering if you have the strength to carry it through to the end.

Your commitment must be *to a plan of action* that will see you expending at least two hundred calories more each day as soon as you build the physical capacity to do so. To dream of some goal several months down the line with no clear and feasible plan for achieving it is to court disaster once again.

Most people start a weight loss program with a statement such as "I am going to lose x pounds by such and such a date." Then, they undertake some drastic diet and/or frenzied exercise routine that they hate and can stick with for only a short period of time. That is not the plan of action and commitment I am talking about.

In the last chapter I gave an example of how making some small but significant change in your behavior immediately upon getting up in the morning feeds back into your mental processes and forces a change in your self-concept. If you arise with the intention of doing the first minute of an exercise routine, with a plan of how you are going to build it up to ten or fifteen minutes, and then carry out your intention, you illustrate willpower and commitment. The successful action reinforces your commitment and the strength of your commitment grows with success.

So, you start with a commitment to a rational plan for increasing walking (or some other aerobic activity of your choice). If at first you do not see how you can make the slightest change in your life, then you must complete the life management exercise I describe in chapter seven. When you have selected the time for your activity and have it firmly in mind or written on your daily calendar, its completion will increase the strength of your resolve. In time, the joy of being active will take over and you will no longer feel any motivational conflict.

But unfortunately, in the early stages there is a problem getting your new activities imprinted in the fabric of your life. It may take six months, and possibly a year, to make physical activity so important to you that nothing takes priority over it during its scheduled time. It often takes a full year for a person to work out a life-long activity program because *it must fit all seasons.*

Here is an example of what may happen. Three winters back we had a great snowfall in Nashville. It caused the cancellation of classes in public schools and at the university. When schools close, we postpone weight group meetings to avoid confusion and travel problems. I had a tennis match scheduled that day at an indoor tennis facility. I have studded snow tires and can get around in most Nashville snow storms. I decided first to drop by one of the large health spas to see what was going on. It was jammed—people who did not have to go to work were jogging around the indoor track, lined up six deep at the weight machines, and overflowing the swimming pool. I drove to the Y a few blocks away; it was equally as crowded. I could not find a parking place. When I arrived at the tennis center, I inquired whether any courts were open after my singles match, since my partner and I wanted to join some others for doubles. Not one court was available until closing time at 11 P.M.

In all my journey, observing at least two hundred people in action that day, only one was obviously fat.

When the weight group met the following week, I asked how many people had kept their activity level up during the storm. *Not one!*

Why? Because the weather was bad!

For too many fat people it is always too hot, too cold, raining, snowing, or hay fever season.

But not for thin people who love to be active.

That is one reason why the probationary period for building

activity into your life can last a year. You have to be committed enough to devise—and sometimes invest in—an activity program that you can carry out all year long.

Fat people do not find it easy to walk or jog in the snow. And for sure, if you are seriously overweight it is harder to get around. But when it snows, committed walkers and joggers cannot wait to get out to experience the special thrill that accompanies laying down the first footprints in the fresh white blanket that covers their favorite routes.

Once you lose weight and get fit, you will have joined that group and will never get fat again.

So, commitment to change must be renewed in the face of environmental pressures and old habits that tend to push you back to square one.

Commitment to change can be renewed by making each sign of success prominent in your consciousness and in your environment. You must seize every opportunity to change what may be a defeatist attitude and reward yourself for every beneficial change in your behavior.

Start talking to yourself, giving yourself a verbal pat on the back for every single successful minute of change. It illustrates willpower and it illustrates commitment.

Make the record of your successes visible to yourself and to others. For example, some people keep a cumulative graph of their daily walking mileage posted conspicuously at home or at work. If graphs confuse you, just use a page from a yearly calendar and jot down your mileage each day. Many people find that posting such a graph or calendar on the refrigerator door is much more rewarding and encouraging than having a fat picture of themselves posted there for all to see. That walking record is something to be proud of.

Lack of family support and friendly cooperation can help to undermine all but the strongest resolution. In order to carry out your intentions to increase activity, you may have to negotiate time with husband or wife, children, roommate, and relatives. Just stand firm: *we all deserve each other's help to find the time to be fit.* As part of the life management exercise, I describe how to plan the family responsibility and activity calendar. This technique has helped many overworked homemakers and business people organize the family into an active support system.

Beginning walkers often want and need company. When you become an experienced walker you may discover that walking by yourself is equally or even more gratifying than social walking. To begin, when you feel the need for company, you can organize your neighborhood, church group, social club, or business colleagues into a walking group. Put up signs, publish announcements in your church or social group bulletins, call your friends, or just put a note like the following in twenty mail boxes in your neighborhood. It has helped a number of people, especially women, organize neighborhood walking groups.

I have just started a walking program and I am looking for (male / female) walking companions in our neighborhood. I can walk at (name hours and days) and would really like your company. Please call me at ___ ____ if you are interested.

If you like, you can volunteer to share with your walking buddies the information that you gain from reading this book and others in the fitness area. Soon you will replace your concern with overeating and dieting with new things you are learning and enjoying about being fit.

Reading and Learning

"For the first time in my life I am not obsessed with food." That statement is repeated over and over again by people who have found the fitness route to getting rid of excess fat.

It is time to stop reading about diets and worrying about your eating transgressions. It is time to fill your mind with plans for your next walk, jog, game, dance class, or that vacation which you are going to be much more fit to enjoy.

Active people read about their favorite sports and activities. If they want to learn yoga and try out some new postures, they read a book or two, and possibly enroll in a class. The same with strength training, aerobic dance, tennis, jogging, walking, racquet ball, and anything else connected with activity. They stop paying attention to the newest miracle diets that appear in the monthly magazines. They finally appreciate how useless these diets prove to be.

It is not that active people lose interest in nutrition. Many report studying nutrition more carefully than ever before, but their purpose is to learn in order to enhance their health and their ability in their chosen activity. No more crash diets, even if they want to lose a few pounds. They know such diets are not healthful and most likely will only reduce the energy they need for their activities.

To help fill your mind with the kind of productive thoughts that active people entertain about themselves and their body, you can start by reading one book each week on some fitness topic. Then you can begin to experiment with some of the suggestions in your own active life.

I have listed a few books on walking, jogging, tennis, bicycling, strength training, and yoga, as well as some on the general topic of physical fitness in the bibliography. Replace some of your other readings or "spectating time" with some readings in these new areas and with more "doing."

When you stop thinking about how difficult it is to diet and start filling your mind with the things that active people think about, your mental contents will begin to support your new lifestyle.

Fantasy

As valuable as reading can be, however, the most valuable mental contents are those that you create for yourself. This book and any other can only point the way and tell you what other people have in their heads. You may ruminate a little on the ideas of others, but until these ideas become translated into your own personal vocabulary, experienced in your own body, and felt in your own moving muscles, they cannot motivate you. Other people's fantasies belong to them. You cannot see what they saw and feel what they felt as they write about them.

But reading what others have written *can* stimulate you to free your own mental processes. They *can* inspire you to create the atmosphere in which your own imaginative faculties can grow. One single powerful image (like the fighter image that paved the way for Cindy's success), an image that may hit you when you least expect it, can turn the tide once and for all in your favor.

Here is an example of imagery at work. It occurred while walking and helped insure the success of another formerly fat man.

I was out early one morning after I had been in the program for about two months. I was doing pretty good in my walking—not perfect, but maybe five days a week. I had lost about twenty pounds and I could feel the difference. I started going faster. I got this impulse to go as fast as I could.

That is when I got this picture in my mind. First, I began to feel how strong my legs were. I looked down and watched my legs as I moved. I remember feeling pleased with how the shape of my legs had changed. I was beginning to sweat. I thought about my footsteps. In each step I was leaving a little bit of fat behind me.

I know sweat isn't body fat, but sweating made me think of droplets of body fat. I saw my footsteps behind me and little droplets of fat in each footstep. I thought to myself, "I'm moving out"—like a race car burning rubber, or maybe a race horse kicking up the dirt behind him—and I thought to myself, "I'm leaving fat behind me."

I still think about this even now, sometimes when I'm out running, especially if I think I ate too much last night.

Here is another bit of imagery which I have suggested to others because it helped me eat a little bit less when I wanted to see how I would feel five pounds lighter about a year ago.

There were two things you said that helped me a lot. One was how, when I felt hungry, it was my fat cells sending me a message that I was losing weight. They were urging me to eat so that they could stay big and fat. I began to think how good that feeling of being hungry was, instead of how bad! The other was to concentrate on how my body felt when I was walking and jogging. I thought about how my stomach was getting smaller and flatter.

I always walked or jogged in the morning on an empty stomach, so I was always at my flattest and thinnest then. As I was going down the road, I would think of how I would feel if I weighed a few pounds less—how much lighter, stronger, and faster I would be. I would imagine I was already like that. I could feel it. Then, several times during the day I would think about how I felt that morning when I was running.

I used it as a way to help me stop stuffing myself at night. Before dinner I would think for a minute of how I felt walking and jogging earlier that day, and how I wanted to feel. Then I could eat slowly and stop before I was full up to my ears.

By using fantasy and body movement appropriately, you can take some deliberate steps to develop new attitudes and feelings, and a new set of personality characteristics. Certain body movements have an intrinsic meaning that feeds back into your psychological experience. And the way you think about yourself and your body movements can reinforce self-directed psychological changes. It may sound complicated, but it isn't. Here is how it works.

If you have never done this experiment, do it now. Break into a big smile. Notice how you feel? Now erase the smile and frown. See the difference?

In miniature, this experiment demonstrates how neuromuscular feedback can influence mood. Along similar lines, other research demonstrates how learning to reduce muscle tension can feed back into your consciousness and reduce the experience of anxiety. To sample this effect, take a deep breath—hold it for a moment—now let it out as you loosen tension in your shoulder area. Consciously feel the relaxation. This little exercise actually slowed your heart rate momentarily a few beats per minute because your rate of respiration and level of muscle tension have physiological feedback connections to your heart. With practice, using a variety of techniques under conscious control, people have learned to alter blood pressure, brain waves, heart rate, body temperature, and other bodily processes that may affect their mood and physical well-being.

To experience fully, easily, and not just momentarily, how your mind and body interact to change feelings, attitudes, and even basic personality characteristics, practice the following mental and physical exercise several times. It will have immediate direct effects. But of greater importance, it will stimulate you to develop your own way of putting your mind and body together to be the kind of person you want to be.

First, one day as you are walking, ask yourself, "How does a proud, strong, self-confident person walk?" Then, walk that way for at least five minutes. Examine your feelings and see what you change about your walking style. Because this is new, you may have to exaggerate at first, so really get into it and be the proudest, strongest, most self-confident person in this world, and translate these characteristics into your walking style.

Second, reverse the process. Start with the body, forget mental attitude, and give no psychological label to anything you do. Just lengthen your stride and pick up the pace slightly. Let your feet strike the ground firmly, but push off lightly with your toes. Let your arms swing freely. Fix your gaze on some distant point about eye level, but at least several blocks ahead of you. Square your shoulders and lengthen your body. Watch that distant point. You will feel very tall. Do this for five minutes and reflect on your feelings and thoughts.

As the spirit moves you, switch back and forth, from the mental initiation of the walking style to any physical style you desire that does not have any preconceived mental implications.

On the mental side, project a variety of attitudes, feelings, or personal characteristics into your body movement. Become the person you want to be as you walk. To get you started, here is a partial list of self-descriptive adjectives with different shades of meaning that can be translated into your walking style. They can be translated into other body movements as well. Try them out.

independent	proud	relaxed
self-reliant	self-confident	vigorous
persistent	graceful	light
intent	fearless	dynamic
assertive	committed	strong
fresh	happy	talented
attractive	disciplined	tough
thin	courageous	

For some interesting variety, try fantasizing the characteristics of animals whose movements or temperaments seem interesting. I know walkers and runners who "become" birds, leopards, gazelles, cats, greyhound dogs, or German shepherds; I know one man who likes to be a bear.

When you reverse to an emphasis on your physical side, experiment with variations in stride, long steps or short, gliding or bouncing; hold your arms high or low, pumping or dangling them as you go up hills; head high, head low; and, of course, variations in speed. Avoid, however, anything that increases muscle tension and produces unnecessary strain in your movements for any length of time.

Enter fully into this exercise for an experience you may remember for a lifetime. *But do not feel that you must repeat it any specified number of times.* Let your reactions guide you. In the end you will develop your own way of relating physical and mental experience.

I said at the beginning of this section that the fantasies, images, and strategies of others belong to them, not you. The experiment above is designed to get you started and to illustrate the striking way in which mind and body can work together to make changes. As you begin to read in the fitness area, you will come across some of the fantasies and experiences that inspire people willing to write about them—your everyday jogger, as well as your world class athletes.

However, when I talk with successful weight losers, and walkers and runners for whom physical activity is so rewarding, I find that it is the spontaneous, unexpected fantasies and images which arise out of their personal dreams and life experience that have the most dramatic and lasting impact. The kind of imagery and fantasy I mean only occurs when you are out on a long walk or jog, alone with your own thoughts.

If you pursue the discipline I suggest and build to that forty to sixty minutes a day of some steady state aerobic activity, your own mind will, one day, without warning, break away from its customary channels.

In contrast with the planned experiment I have just described, you need not do anything in particular with your mental processes to free them. In fact, the less you try, the more likely you are to generate something previously hidden in the depth of your own being that has a meaning you will feel in every cell of your body. All you can and need do is set the stage for this to happen. The stage is set when you swing your body into the rhythmic motion of a long walk or jog and let your mind do what it will.

When you walk with strength and confidence, I think you will find that the feelings in your body will stick with you throughout your days and generalize to other situations. It will help you deal with anything that comes your way. Many people have written that walking or jogging has somehow helped them solve their most difficult problems. People in my weight groups make similar statements. Although being physically fit and enjoying the psychological benefits that go along with the process may not solve any problems in a direct way, it certainly seems to make people feel that they are more competent to live productively and to deal with adversity when necessary.

The Ultimate Benefit

You have heard this statement before: "I cannot imagine anyone walking or jogging four or five miles at a time. Isn't it boring?"

No.

Only to the uninitiated.

Each of us has led a life rich and unique in experience. There is in each of us a repository of talents and ideas unduplicated in any other person living or dead. But we never take the time to get to know ourselves. When we pay attention to our thoughts and feelings, it is often hurried and under pressure. We allow ourselves to be at the mercy of every outside influence—always responding to the telephone or the knock on our office door, always fulfilling the responsibilities of work and family. We are continually being distracted. We rarely develop into the persons we can or want to be.

When you reach the point where walking or jogging for forty-five minutes or more becomes effortless and you have allowed your imagination and thoughts to roam freely, you will get to know yourself in a qualitatively different way. You will grow to like yourself more than you have ever thought possible. I am not speaking about ego or conceit when I say this.

You will discover that you are your own best friend and most interesting companion. That is the ultimate benefit of distance walking and jogging. It is an incomparable experience.

I could elaborate at great length on what this transformation means to people who have talked with me about it and others who have written about it. It would be words again, however, and not your own experience. The only way to really know what I mean is for you to enter into the discipline that can make this experience a reality.

Start walking.

7

STOP KIDDING YOURSELF—
YOU HAVE THE TIME

Working Out Your Daily Schedule

If you have any doubts about your ability to reorganize your life to reach your new weight loss and fitness goals, here is a way to remove them. I have yet to meet the person who keeps a daily record of what he or she has done on the half hour for a full week, who can honestly say "there is no time" to make changes.

If you cannot mentally review your daily schedule and immediately come up with specific times for some physical activity, monitor your life for at least a week. In a small notebook or on a lined pad, record in the format suggested here what you do on the half hour. Some people recall everything, once each day, filling in the daily record just before they go to sleep each night. Others pause three times, at lunch, dinner, and just before they go to bed, to complete the record. This leads to greater accuracy.

In the comments column, jot down whether the behaviors you record at each time are what you planned and wanted to do, and whether you want to continue doing them. Some people also record the mood that was associated with their actions throughout the day. This may help you discover how your affects and actions are related. The record will alert you to what you want to change and where you can substitute some activity for one of your present behaviors.

I schedule between one and two hours a day in some sport or physical activity. You do not have to do that much to be healthy, fit, and slim. I do it because I like to.

When I became Chairman of the Department of Psychology in

Monitor of Daily Activity

	Activity	Comments
6:00 A.M.		
6:30		
7:00		
7:30		
8:00		
8:30		
9:00		
9:30		
10:00		
10:30		
11:00		
11:30		
Noon		
12:30 P.M.		
1:00		
1:30		
2:00		
2:30		
3:00		
3:30		
4:00		
4:30		
5:00		
5:30		
6:00		
6:30		
7:00		
7:30		
8:00		
8:30		
9:00		
9:30		
10:00		
10:30		
11:00		
11:30		
Midnight		

1970, I sent a memo to the faculty. Among other things, it informed them that I would be out of the office every afternoon for two hours playing tennis. I promised that I would find time during the rest of the day for appointments and for any other responsibilities as chairman.

One of my colleagues came to my office, slammed his fist down on my desk and asked, "Dick, do you mean playing tennis is more important than being department chairman?" "Of course," I replied. "If I have to give up tennis to be chairman, you can take the job and shove it!"

There was plenty of time during the day for everything, but to this day, my walk, jog, or tennis match goes down on my daily calendar first. I can still work twelve hours a day or more whenever necessary.

Several years later, the colleague who questioned me became as much of a sports enthusiast as I. He runs and plays racquet ball on a regular basis.

Do you have to have academic freedom to live this kind of a life? Of course not. I have worked with busy executives, professional people, and those who push time clocks. They, too, can do what we have done. True, some people have to drop coffee breaks, or a portion of their television time, or that quick stop at the cocktail lounge on the way home from work, for a walk or tennis match. Some are walking or bicycling to and from work. If you have a secretary who makes appointments for you, get him or her to enter your walk, jog, tennis match, or gym time *every day each week*, before anything else is entered. It will soon become the most important appointment in your day. With that walk or active game on your schedule, you will be well on your way to successful weight management.

The Family Calendar

The greatest scheduling problems occur in families with children where both parents work. Men generally find it easy to inform their families of their new plans and the families fall in line. Unfortunately, the women do not find it equally as simple. The working wife usually still retains most, if not all, of the typical mother functions: car pools, doctors' appointments, chauffering children after

THE FAMILY CALENDAR

Family tasks: who does what with whom and when.
Everyone helps everyone else get at least forty-five minutes for activity

	Mon.	Tue.	Wed.	Thur.	Fri.	Sat.	Sun.
6:00 A.M.							
7:00							
8:00							
9:00							
10:00							
11:00							
Noon							
1:00 P.M.							
2:00							
3:00							
4:00							
5:00							
6:00							
7:00							
8:00							
9:00							
10:00							
11:00							
Midnight							

school to extracurricular activities, and most of the daily household tasks.

Of course, many men and women know how to share these responsibilities. But unfortunately, many do not. The women are so accustomed to being mother and housewife in the traditional sense that they feel they must still continue with all of these responsibilities in spite of a full-time outside job.

Male or female, if you are having trouble finding time to be active and feel that your work and family responsibilities are so great that nothing can be done to change the situation, do not give up yet.

Sit down in a full-family conference and inform everyone that you are all going to have to work together to make at least forty-five minutes available to you as your very own. Lay out on a large sheet a family calendar in the format illustrated. For every hour of the day, enter on this one large sheet what everyone in the family wants to do and needs to do for an entire week. Indicate how the needs will be met: who needs to do what, when, and with whom. You expect the collaboration of your family in making at least forty-five minutes available to you; you, in turn, expect to collaborate with them in reaching their objectives.

I think we all have some sense of fairness and justice. In families that care for each other, this kind of strategy always works. In fact, the major stumbling block for fat women is that they frequently are so used to being martyrs they find it difficult to get comfortable with this new freedom when it is offered. Give yourself a chance. You can get used to it!

The Executive Walk

Here are two techniques that I have suggested to those driven executives who feel they cannot take a minute off from work for walking. Although I feel the mind and body need an activity time out, there may be some days when work piles up and you need to get some letters off or make notes for an upcoming meeting.

I have done considerable work while walking and jogging. While walking I sometimes carry a hand-sized tape recorder with an automatic sound level control. It has a pause button on top and a wrist strap to prevent dropping. I can dictate letters, make lecture notes, or outline a research strategy for one of our weight management studies. My secretary has become expert in typing from this dictation in spite of my heavier breathing and the slight background traffic noise. When I interrupted one dictation to ask her if she found it troublesome, she answered, "No. I only wish I, too, could be out there with you instead of being indoors typing!"

I have other simple techniques for jogging and walking that will allow you to store ideas for future use, or for writing a lecture or article. Walkers can carry a pocket-sized pad or a few sheets of blank paper folded in their pockets. Both walkers and runners can use a well-known mnemonic device called a *pegword list*. This involves making a visual association between an object or idea in your mind with the image in the pegword list. I assure you that if you use such a device, when you get back to your office, your recall will be perfect.

Here is the list:

One is a bun, two is a shoe, three is a tree, four is a door, five is a hive, six is sticks, seven is heaven, eight is a gate, nine is wine, ten is a hen.

Try using this list for those groceries you will need to get started on the Double Your Fat Loss Diet (chapter ten) to get the hang of it. For example, put the hamburger meat inside the bun and visualize it. A hunk of cheese can fit inside the shoe, hang your vegetables from the tree, plaster the eggs on the door. The images will stick with you as long as you need them, or until you use the list another day.

When I use the list for writing or for preparing a speech, I put some visual representation of an idea I wish to remember with a pegword object. *The most absurd or ridiculous connections are the easiest to recall.*

If you have more than ten ideas or objects, circle the list twice. The images will remain separate because the second image attached to the bun acts as a marker for the second go-around. However, you will probably never need to go around twice to recall the things you want from an hour's walk or jog. You may with a grocery list.

When problems that stubbornly elude solution beset you, a working walk can sometimes be a very exciting and creative experience. Just quit beating your head against the wall and let the mind wander the first fifteen or twenty minutes. It loosens. If you have been rigidly pursuing a line of thought that leads to a dead end, cracks will appear in that rigidity. Novel ideas will trickle through. If you get a rush of ideas, be sure to store them with your pegword list or use that pocket-size notebook you can carry with you. There is nothing more frustrating than returning to your office with a gaping hole in your line of thought and have to struggle to fill it. I know of one runner who had a great idea while running down a dirt road. He stopped and wrote out several words in the dirt and jogged on, thinking about other things. He did indeed find that he could not quite recall his line of thought, so he drove back to the spot. Unfortunately, car tracks had obliterated his notes.

Try holding all two-person business meetings "on the road." There is no reason why two people need to sit and talk when they can walk and talk. This becomes the two-person executive walk. You will come to like your associates more, close better deals, reach more amicable solutions to problems, and contribute to your colleagues' health and well-being. Walking can raise your spirits, clear your heads, and put you in a better frame of mind for working together. Well-oxygenated brains work best.

EQUIPMENT FOR WALKING

Shoes and Clothing

The only essential equipment for walking that may not be in the beginning walker's wardrobe is a pair of good walking shoes. Jogging shoes usually work better than anything else for city and light country walking. Some manufacturers are introducing new styles especially for walkers. Do not skimp in the care expended or the cost when you purchase your shoes: try on a variety, walk around the store, be sure they do not slip around the heel, and do not pinch the toes. I strongly advise you to shop at specialty stores that cater to walkers and joggers. The salespersons at such stores will know their merchandise well. They will appreciate your need to test the shoes, even to go out around the block. Do it. Shop on a clear dry day so that you can give your shoes a good test. Remember, the slightest rub along an edge or across a seam can mean a blister a mile or two down the road.

When you shop for shoes, wear the same style socks you will be using when walking. Many walkers like a thick 100 percent wool or cotton sock. Some long-distance walkers use a thin cotton under a thick woolen sock, but I know some walkers and runners who wear no socks at all. For years I have used thick synthetic fiber athletic socks, soft to the touch. A combination such as 80 percent orlon and 20 percent cotton or nylon is, for me, satisfactorily absorbent and longer lasting than the more expensive woolens. While I find it possible to save a little on atheltic socks, I always buy the very best fitting shoes no matter what the cost.

Daily walkers and joggers like to vary shoes from day to day.

Most own at least two pairs. If you begin to cover long distances, you, too, may find that this is a strategy that reduces the likelihood of aches and pains. A variety of shoes will spread some of the stress of walking among the different muscles involved. There are many good brands, but because I do a lot of walking and running on asphalt, I like a well-cushioned shoe such as the Brooks Vantage, and the New Balance 420. The Brooks Vantage seems especially suited to people with a wide hip structure. The inner edge of the heel is raised a few degrees. This elevation compensates, somewhat, for the angle at which the foot of the wide-hipped person strikes the pavement. However, some people find this style uncomfortable after several miles of walking. Brooks makes other styles which I have not yet tried, including a walker. The New Balance feels especially good on very long walks or jogs. This brand offers a narrow as well as standard width. Many walkers like the Nike, Adidas, and Puma brands. Since shoe styles and construction techniques are changing frequently, ask the shoe salesperson what seems to be working out best for the use you plan.*

As for the rest of your apparel, the lighter the better. You will warm up as you go along and if you dress too heavily you will be shedding clothes along the route. It is better to dress in several light layers rather than one or two heavier ones. This way, if you wish to shed something, you can tie it around your waist. The only exception I make to the "travel light" advice is when you have a muscular ache or pain. Under those conditions you will want to go a bit slower and keep warm. It may call for an extra layer.

One piece of clothing has been invaluable to me. It is a light, closely woven, unlined nylon shell that you can purchase at an Army–Navy surplus store for about five dollars. Mine has a hood, but still weighs only a few ounces. This item can cost up to twenty or thirty dollars in fine sporting goods stores, but I can not imagine one at any price serving any better than mine. These shells are water resistant, not waterproof. While they breathe slightly, they are perfect for resisting the wind and helping your inner layers of clothing preserve your body heat. I have run in calm fair weather as low as five degrees Fahrenheit with a thermal underwear top, a

---

*The company making Brooks shoes has been sold to Wolverine, Inc. You may need to look for shoes in the Brooks style under a new name in 1982.

cotton flannel shirt, and the shell over both with perfect comfort. In a cold wind, I would add another layer. If you are going to walk or run consistently in cold weather, be sure to own one or two medium weight woolen sweaters. Wool is best for preserving body heat even when wet from rain or perspiration, as I know from personal experience.

Once, running in winter on a strange trail in the Great Smokies, I found myself jogging across an exposed mile-long ridge. The wind and temperature together yielded a chill factor of at least minus fifteen degrees below zero. I was thankful I had that woolen sweater and my nylon shell on top of a couple of light cotton layers.

You can find medium weight woolen sweaters at discount houses for twenty dollars or less. Don't worry about the dry cleaning instructions. Use Woolite and lay the sweater out over a towel or bathtub rack to dry. Drying may take two days, which is why I have two of them.

In winter you will want to keep your head, ears, and hands warm as well as your feet. I like the thick woven ski or stocking caps, and I wear socks over my hands rather than gloves or mittens—on really cold days, two pairs. If the snow is several inches high or wet, I use hiking boots with vibram soles for traction. But if the snow is light and fresh and the temperature below freezing, regular jogging shoes are by far the best. The snow will not melt on your shoes and they will not soak through. On very cold days I use two pairs of socks on my feet as well as my hands.

Most walkers and joggers don't like to have their legs encumbered on really brisk walks or fast runs, and, in cold weather, it is not as important for heat preservation to cover your legs as it is your head, torso, hands, and feet. However, for walking at a moderate pace most of my walking friends like a warm-up suit when the temperature dips into the fifties, especially if they plan a stop or two along the way. I don't climb into warm-up pants for jogging until the temperature gets below forty degrees. If I'm going on a fast run, I won't wear them until it gets below freezing.

In summer I suggest you avoid the heat of the day for walking or jogging, but if you must go out, try a white floppy tennis hat over your head. I find it keeps me much more comfortable than going bare-headed.

Once I went for a training jog in ninety-five degree temperature with two friends who were preparing for a race that was sure to be held in similar heat two days later. This is not a wise thing to do for anyone, no matter what his condition. But we are not always wise. I filled a plastic baggie with ice, wrapped it in paper towels, and stuck it in my tennis hat, which I tied to my head with a long shoelace. Two miles down the road my friends were near collapse, while I was cool and comfortable. I took off my hat, poured part of the cold water from the melted ice over their heads and shoulders, and let them drink the rest. We decided to limit our jog to four slow miles that day.

Never let a light rain deter you from a walk. Do, of course, avoid electrical storms. They are dangerous. Some of your greatest walks and jogs will take place in the rain, however. Some people use standard rain apparel with well-placed air holes to allow some breathing of the inner layers of clothing. These air vents are usually placed under the arms and under a flap across the back. Other walkers prefer the light rainsuits that joggers use (forty to eighty dollars and very comfortable). Except in cold weather I never bother with special rainwear for jogging. But when it's windy and chilly, as well as raining, I use a waterproof jacket over whatever extra underlayers I think advisable. This jacket was another five-dollar item at the Army–Navy surplus store.

Since I have several pairs of jogging shoes, I do not mind soaking one pair for the joy of a forty-five-minute walk or jog in the rain. I never bother with rubbers. Dry your shoes with newspapers stuffed inside, or if they have nylon or canvas uppers, you can throw them in a dryer on low heat.

It will take trial and error to find out what is best for you in the various extremes of weather. You may not pick the perfect attire on your first attempts—but don't let that deter you from starting out. I still recall trying to make up my mind about what I should wear before starting out to jog in the rain for the first time. It was early in the morning one spring day, with the temperature forty-two degrees. After about five minutes of debate about whether to wear a warm-up suit, whether to try out my waterproof jacket for the first time, and how many layers I should wear, I found I was getting tense and irritable over what usually is a fun activity. I suddenly realized that my concern was totally unnecessary. If I chose the wrong clothing, it wouldn't be the end of the world. I could turn around and come home. So, I chose light—no warm up pants, just jogging shorts, one cotton flannel over my T shirt, and the waterproof jacket. How fortunate. About twenty minutes out, the rain stopped. A few minutes later the clouds broke and the rays from the early morning sunrise streamed through. I opened the waterproof jacket to let the air circulate and had one of the most memorable hours of jogging in my life.

So, don't spend time worrying about your clothing choices when you start experimenting. Adhere to the fundamental principle: the faster you expect to walk or jog, the lighter you should dress. If your choice doesn't work out the first time, you will be wiser and ready for the second. Once you have cycled the seasons, you will be ready for anything.

When walking or jogging becomes an essential activity in your life, you will want to hit the trails in the woods and hills for some glorious moments that cannot be duplicated anywhere else. You may also get the urge for some all-day or even overnight hikes. Then it is time to branch out and read some of the books I suggest in the bibliography. These discuss special equipment for all sorts of weather and trail conditions. They will tell you where to write for information on walking throughout the country.

Pedometers

With walking becoming more popular, several varieties of pedometers have appeared on the market, including some electronic gadgets with rather high price tags. I suggest you examine the mechanical one distributed by the Pedo Company called the *Precise Pedometer,* as well as any of the other models available at sporting goods stores and large department stores such as Sears Roebuck. They retail around fifteen dollars.

I personally prefer the Precise because it has an easy-to-adjust stride measurement, registers to twenty-five miles before it begins to recircle its easy-to-read dial, and is simple to reset to zero. Unlike some other models, you cannot erase its register by mistake. Although the reading on the stride adjustment scale may not end up corresponding to the actual length of your stride, once you have fussed with the pedometer and gotten it to be correct over a quarter-mile distance, you can count on its accuracy on reasonably level terrain. Mine is right on the button over a measured five-mile distance, but I must set the stride for two and a half feet when I am actually striding closer to three. No matter what I do trying to compensate in the stride adjustment, I cannot get other mechanical models to operate as accurately as the Precise. The company also handles a model especially for joggers. This style, called The Jogger, requires the impact of the running foot to operate. The stride adjustment goes up to six feet.

The Precise has two minor drawbacks: the plastic case may crack if you bend over and the pedometer gets caught in the bend at your waist, and it breaks easily when dropped. However, the company backs up its warranty 100 percent. If you don't tamper with the pedometer and it breaks, the company replaces it with a brand new one for a small postage and handling fee. It's nice to know you can count on them. Keep the package it comes in, with the warranty, in case you have to send it back.

Is it worth buying one? Yes, even though you may stop wearing it all the time after a few weeks or months. It's a motivational aid at first, and will tell you how much you walk in your daily tasks as well as on your special forty-five-minute jaunts. After a while you may reserve its use for your weekend hikes. I have all my patients wear one to determine what their baselines really are. Most continue to wear them for months to be sure they add another three miles a day when their usual daily activities give them only two. Once you wear one it will open your eyes to the small amount of walking your life requires.

One of my patients insisted she walked a mile while shopping forty-five minutes at the grocery. I told her it was more like one-quarter mile. She wanted to make a small wager with me but I wouldn't take it. I already knew from many measurements that most supermarket tours require very little walking. She was surprised to find I was right in her case too. In another instance, a waitress told me that she was sure her job required five or six miles of walking a day. That sounded reasonable to me, too. But her pedometer told her three. That puzzled both of us until we figured out that it would take sixty-six round trips from the counter where she picked up her orders to her *farthest* assigned table forty feet away to make one mile. Since her closest table was only about fifteen feet away, she was indeed making hundreds of trips back and forth each day to equal that three miles. The record keeping, however, made her aware that outside of the breakfast and lunch hours, she spent most of her time sitting and chatting with the other employees.

The Walking Stick and Safety Aids

A few of my walking friends carry a walking stick. Some walkers enjoy collecting them. They can afford protection against man and beast. You can play games and do exercises with them along the route. I frequently meet one confirmed walker in my favorite Nashville park who carries his infant girl in one arm as he exercises with two golf clubs tied together in the other. His little girl can't walk very far on her own, so he alternates clubs and child from arm to arm. You can get quite a workout in forty-five minutes that way.

The walking stick (it can be a tree branch just for carrying) makes you feel better if you are fearful of dogs. However, your best approach with dogs is sweet talk. No matter how angry the animal may seem to you, it's usually just protecting its territory. When you are in the road, or cross to the other side of the street, you are out of the dog's territory and it knows it. Your sweetest "that's a good doggie" intoned like a broken record will do the trick.

But you may want to keep a more aggressive technique in reserve just in case. Dogs do a lot of bluffing, just to see who's going to be the boss. They do it with each other to establish a dominance hierarchy and they do it with people. You can play the same game and win except with animals that are truly vicious and trained to attack. That's where the walking stick comes in handy. Once when I was traveling in Arkansas, I scouted some back forest roads I wished to run. I discovered a pack of three dogs belonging to a farmer along the way. They charged my van as I passed. That concerned me, even though I knew they were not wild. When I ran the route (it passed a scenic bluff overlooking the Arkansas river), I picked up a hefty branch a few hundred yards before I neared that house. When the dogs charged I held the branch like a spear, lifted it high in the air above my head, growled back, and shouted in my most commanding voice, "Go home!" The dogs stopped dead in their tracks and did their barking from a distance.

One of my walking friends swears that red pepper sprinkled on your shoes and pressed into the seams will definitely deter all dogs. I have not tried that technique.

If you know there is a vicious dog in your neighborhood, don't be unnecessarily brave. Dogs do occasionally bite. There is no need to walk scared. Contact the owner, call the dog pound, do whatever it takes to make your route safe and pleasurable. If necessary, *learn to use and carry an aerosol gas repellant or a water pistol filled fifty-fifty with ammonia and water.* One spray will do it forever. Dogs have excellent memories.

Don't stop walking.

9

SENSIBLE DIETING

Why Diet?

"Dieting? I thought you recommend activity as the ultimate solution to the obesity problem. Why do you recommend any diet at all? Why is your dieting/activity program better than any other approach?"

Let's take each point, one at a time.

Although sensible dieting facilitates weight loss, activity *is* the ultimate solution. You would lose an honest thirty pounds of fat (not water weight that comes back) in one year if you began today with my activity program and didn't change your eating habits. At the end of the year you might have to eat more than you do now to stop yourself from losing. Between the direct energy requirements of forty-five minutes a day of any activity equivalent to brisk walking plus the general elevation of metabolic rate resulting from such activity, you will burn up over 100,000 calories from your fat stores in one year. When you decide to stop losing, that level of activity *prevents* 100,000 calories—that's about thirty pounds of fat—from being put back into your fat stores every single year. So I repeat, activity is the ultimate solution and forty-five minutes per day is within the reach of everyone.

So, why diet at all? And if you do diet, how do you avoid the dangers of dieting I've been warning against?

Through activity alone you can expect to lose about two-thirds of a pound of real fat a week. It is still healthful for most people to lose at double that rate or a little faster—one and a half to two pounds a week—through diet and activity. And most people find that it is much more satisfying to get thirty pounds of fat permanently off in fifteen to twenty weeks than to take a full year. The average person will, in that short period, lose thirty pounds of fat (*plus* a few pounds of water in the first week) with my Double Your Fat Loss Diet.

There are other reasons for combining diet with activity. Most sedentary people cannot and should not immediately jump to a full forty-five minutes of activity each day. In addition, it is advisable to begin activity at low intensity levels. It may take you several weeks to reach an average of forty-five minutes a day and if you are walking, a moderate three miles per hour pace is recommended. When you can do forty-five minutes comfortably at that pace, you can begin to speed up, but it may be several more weeks before you can do a large percentage of your walking at three and a half or four miles per hour. Thus, because it is best to begin activity slowly, it will be several weeks before you reach the point where you can comfortably burn two-thirds of a pound of fat per week. This makes reliance on activity alone as a weight loss strategy inefficient compared with a combined approach. It is also very encouraging to feel a quicker acquisition of speed, strength, and endurance in one's preferred activity which occurs when weight loss proceeds at a faster rate, with the help of a sensible diet.

To speed the weight loss process, you add relatively high calorie dieting to your program. When you follow my recommendations, both as to amount of food *and* its composition, you avoid all of those dangers of low calorie dieting I have previously spoken about. By cutting back no more than 500 calories a day from your present weight maintenance level (not below 1200 for a woman or 1500 for a man)* you are not likely to experience the drastic metabolic cutback of low calorie dieting. Although there is likely to be some adaptive reduction of one's normal metabolic rate on any diet that leads to weight loss, it will nowhere approach the amount you might experience on a diet of 1000 calories per day or less. However, whatever the degree of metabolic slowdown, an increase in activity plays an extremely important role in facilitating your weight loss. The increase in activity will both offset and counteract the metabolic cutback of dieting. Your activity program will add 10 to 20

---

*I discuss exceptions to this in the case of true slow metabolism problems in chapter twelve.

percent extra energy expenditure each day, offsetting the potential metabolic slowdown should it occur. At the same time, activity combats adaptive metabolic slowdown by actually speeding up your resting metabolic rate as much as 10 percent. This means you may be burning 10 percent more calories while resting or sleeping—simply because you have been active. An increase in metabolism reflects the work your body must do to replace your muscular energy stores and rebuild body tissue for the next day's activity.

The main reason combining activity with diet is so superior to the use of diet alone is that when you reach desirable weight, activity greatly reduces the probability that you will ever get fat again. The success of the weight loss effort is not how much you lose and how fast, but whether you keep it off permanently. Because you are burning up at least 200 calories a day in your activity plus, the added benefits of a slightly higher basal metabolic rate, you can add not only the 500 calories you have cut back on your diet, but approximately 300 calories a day more when you reach desirable weight, and not regain. Unless your eating habits are way out of whack, you are done with dieting forever when you become active.

Body Composition Changes in Dieting and Activity

Any reduction in caloric intake will lead to a water loss. You will get such a loss with my Double Your Fat Loss Diet, but, it will not (I hope) equal the ridiculous claims of the miracle mongers who tantalize you with "as much as twenty pounds off in fourteen days." In one group of forty-four very overweight men and women, we *averaged* nine pounds lost in fourteen days. Because these patients were walking and doing light calisthenics, we know that a much larger percentage of their weight loss was truly fat than would have occurred on a fad or crash diet for the same period of time.

In addition, we also knew that these individuals were in the process of building, not losing, muscle mass. This would help maintain their metabolic rates and their energy levels. But it also means that a true twenty-two pounds of fat loss might only show up as twenty pounds on the scale. Over a two-month period, a person can gain two pounds of muscle tissue. That's good, because it increases basal metabolism and gives you the added strength to make physical activity feel easier and easier.

Combined activity and diet also contributes to a more stable, healthy water balance than can be obtained with diet alone. Even if you suffer from periodic water retention problems, increased activity holds down the amount you retain at such times. Most people do not realize that almost as much moisture is lost through the skin and in breathing each day as is eliminated via the kidneys. By increasing activity, which increases the breathing rate and sweat production, you can help eliminate water retention. You can also help by eating correctly, that is, with naturally diuretic foods such as fresh pineapple, asparagus, greens, and citrus fruits, and by keeping your salt intake low.

A Diet for the Active Weight Loser

The only sound diet for weight loss, weight maintenance, high energy level and all–around health and nutrition is *a high carbo-hydrate* diet!*

That statement comes as a surprise to many veteran dieters— but perhaps that's why they are veterans. In spite of repeated fail-ures, veteran dieters keep on experimenting with unsound diets. Their weights go up and down like a ferris wheel. My objective is to show you how to implement a single successful diet and a style of eating that insures permanent weight control.

A sound diet has several important characteristics. It should (1) provide you with essential nutrients, (2) be interesting and have variety, (3) taste good, (4) be a pleasure to prepare, (5) fit your personal preference for meal planning, (6) have satiety value, and (7) not make such unusual demands that it becomes a burden to follow in and out of your own home. It should not cause you to feel lethargic nor turn your digestive processes topsy-turvy. You

---

*The original Four-S Diet that I invented for my own personal weight loss cam-paign was higher in carbohydrate than it sounds. I ate considerable quantities of fruit and vegetables along with eggs, cheese, lean meat, fish, and fowl. However, it was not a balanced, truly nutritious diet because I almost completely neglected grains. It's fortunate, I believe, that I never dieted for more than four weeks on that plan because I did, on occasion, experience some weakness on the tennis court toward the end of each dieting episode (which is one of the reasons, in addition to my liking for food, that I would only diet for three to four weeks). The diet I recommend here is much safer and healthier than that Four-S plan and it protects you against loss of energy while increasing your activity level.

should not suffer discomfort, get constipated, or experience periods of diarrhea.

To make this diet your last, and establish a new pattern of eating that meets the requirements of a good diet, you need (1) to understand why the principles I recommend are correct, (2) how to make food preparation easy and fun, (3) how to adapt any of your favorite recipes and all styles of food preparation to meet these objectives, (4) how to eat out, and (5) how to whip up meals on the spur of the moment or plan menus for several days in advance and end up healthy either way.

Why High Carbohydrates?

During a period of dieting, you deplete your energy stores of both carbohydrates (sugar in the form of glycogen) and fat. You need some of both to power all of your activities. You have plenty of fat, *but very little glycogen.* Your quick energy stores total about 2000 calories—but every single pound of fat tissue contains 3500 calories. You can deplete your quick energy stores in a matter of hours with vigorous activity, but a person with only twenty pounds of fat has enough stored energy to cover 700 miles of walking if only the energy from fat were required to power that activity. But you become exhausted as soon as you deplete your stored glycogen.

Low calorie, high protein diets really do a job in getting rid of stored glycogen. As I mentioned, this is responsible for a large initial weight loss as well as a substantial gain when you go off such a diet. Such diets can have serious side effects for the active person.

When you get low on stored glycogen, you get low on energy. That is, you feel weak and tired. Indeed you really have considerably less work capacity under these conditions. In contrast, studies have shown that active people on high carbohydrate diets store more glycogen in their muscles (and probably in the liver) and can have up to twice the endurance than when they eat a standard mixed or high fat diet.

If you go on a diet that is *not* high in carbohydrates *and* start an activity program, you may not replace enough glycogen in your quick energy stores each day to keep you feeling zestful and to give you the increasing endurance you are trying to build. You should diet according to the same principles that athletes and coaches use to maintain maximum energy and endurance—you should use a diet high in complex carbohydrates.

As you become active, your muscles are going to learn to store more glycogen because they have that marvelous capacity of adapting to the demands you put on them. You will not be helping this change to occur if you deny them the carbohydrates they need to do the job, and you will not feel as well as you might either.

While the energy availability aspect of our diet is important, a high complex carbohydrate diet has several additional benefits: (1) it provides the fiber essential to smooth digestive processes, (2) it helps *waste* fat; a diet such as I recommend contains enough fiber to combine with up to 100 calories of the fat you eat each day and prevent their absorption, (3) compared with dietary fat, it costs the body four times the amount of energy to put excess carbohydrate calories into your fat stores. It takes about 5 percent of the energy content of dietary fat to convert it to storage. It takes 20 percent of any excess carbohydrates to do the job.

Does a high complex carbohydrate diet go counter to the best available nutritional advice? Not at all.

In 1977, the Select Committee on Nutrition and Human Needs of the United States Senate recommended that as much as 60 percent of the caloric intake be derived from carbohydrates, primarily from vegetables, fruits, and whole grains. Most nutritionists and the medical boards of several countries, including Finland, Norway, and Sweden, make similar recommendations. You only need about 12 percent of your calories from protein, primarily for the repair and regeneration of body tissues. Twenty-five to 30 percent from fat is adequate and satisfying to the palate.

How can a person eat without making a big fuss and many calculations to reach these goals? By learning the simple principles that underlie my Double Your Fat Loss Diet and making some easy changes in food preparation and eating habits.

10

DOUBLE YOUR FAT LOSS DIET

You will lose real fat efficiently, maintain a high energy level, and establish a lifelong pattern of good eating habits by following two simple principles:

1. Eliminate unnecessary fat and sugar from your diet.
2. Increase fruits, vegetables, and whole grains.

By combining an increase in activity with these two dietary principles, almost every obesity problem in the United States would be alleviated, together with many associated health problems.

If you have any poor eating habits, I suspect you are painfully aware of them and have tried to change before. I know it's easy to state simple principles for improvement, but I also know that putting them into practice has been a very different matter.

That is why I have devised a Seven-Day plan to help you learn, step by step, the principles that underlie my Double Your Fat Loss Diet and how to put them into practice. Once you learn the principles, as well as how to select and prepare the foods I suggest, you can either repeat the Seven-Day Plan again and again, or vary it as you please to meet your own food preferences.

Of course one of my objectives is to help you lose weight. Most women who follow the diet plan exactly will lose several pounds the first week and average losing one and a half to two pounds a week thereafter. You do not have to go on and off the diet every two weeks to stay healthy. It averages about 1200 calories a day, which, combined with your activity program should lead to a deficit of between 700 and 1000 calories daily. Men achieve the same deficit with a calorie intake of around 1500 to 1800 calories. They can add more food from all categories, but should concentrate on fruit, vegetables, and grains. The diet already contains enough selections from foods outside these categories to meet nutritional requirements.

In addition to helping you lose weight, however, the Seven-Day Plan is designed with several other important objectives.

General Objectives

1. To illustrate low-fat cooking and eating while showing you how to use just enough fat to preserve the richness of flavor and quality of texture that only fats can provide.

2. To sensitize you to the natural flavors of food and the contribution herb seasoning can make.

3. To teach methods of preparing food that you can enjoy enough to stick with the rest of your life.

4. To teach a simple way of estimating calories so that you will have a feel for caloric content and can make wise choices in any situation.

Because there is so much to learn about nutrition and sensible dieting, it frequently overwhelms people when it is presented in a single large dose. Therefore, I have arranged each day of the plan to provide you with a short lesson to go with some delicious recipes. Each day ends with a review with which you can test yourself to see whether you are following the principles of the diet. By the time you finish the week you will have associated the information with a way of preparing food that affords the kind of taste and variety you can enjoy.

Before you start the diet, read through the entire Seven-Day Plan for an overview. Don't expect to absorb all of the information at once—it will become second nature as you reread and follow the plan each day. You will learn the material better if each day, one day at a time, you explain what you are doing and why to your family or friends.

The Seven-Day Plan begins with a discussion of the breakfast meal. You can select one of a number of basic breakfasts throughout your diet. Specific menus for seven days—lunch and dinner—follow. The chapter concludes with (1) a discussion of the general principles of the Double Your Fat Loss Diet, (2) how to set up a Seven-Day Plan of your own, (3) how to prepare any of your own favorite recipes the low calorie way, (4) how to eat out and still lose weight, (5) the rationale for whole grains in the diet, (6) when, and when not, to use vitamin supplements, (7) why diet drinks can ruin your diet, (8) the use of alcohol, (9) how long to diet, (10) how to insure your success, (11) a simple dietary rule for weight maintenance, and (12) a parcel of superb recipes from my own collection, with a guide to seasonings.

After you have surveyed the entire plan, you can make one of two decisions. You can follow my meal plan exactly, or lay out seven days of your own. But I think you will enjoy everyone of the recipes I suggest in one or another of their variations because I have prepared everyone of them myself many times. I love to cook just as much as I enjoy eating, so I know that in one form or another there is a style of preparation that will fit almost every taste. In addition, each day's menu has been evaluated by expert nutritional consultants for its nutritional value.

Finally, do not start your diet until you complete the Dieter's Checklist which appears later in this chapter. Many people fail in their diets because they don't make adequate preparations to meet all the situations they will encounter in the weeks that follow. The checklist shows you how to set the stage to insure your success.

THE SEVEN-DAY PLAN

The eating plan which follows will provide approximately 1200 calories daily and is appropriate for most women. Men should increase serving sizes by 25 to 50 per cent to provide 1500 to 1800 calories.

The Importance of Breakfast

A very large percentage of fat people skip breakfast. So do thin people. In the case of fat people trying to lose weight, however, it is obviously not working as a weight control strategy. In fact, many overeaters are overeaters as a direct result of skipping breakfast (sometimes, but less frequently lunch). If you do either of these things, there is a great likelihood that you are building up a hidden hunger drive. The drive has a true biological basis. By skipping meals, especially breakfast, you develop a great energy deficit between arising in the morning and your evening meal. It results in raiding your refrigerator or pantry in the late afternoon, or in constant urges to nibble all night long. It forces you to struggle to restrain yourself to a lower caloric intake than your body seems to demand. And once you give in, the flood gates open.

In spite of the fact that their behavior in skipping meals and overeating at night is a perfect illustration of the dangers that arise from exercising too much restraint earlier in the day, many fat people are too frightened to try to change. They feel that once they start to eat, even if it's at breakfast, the flood gates will open just that much sooner. They say to me, "Once I start, I can't stop," and indeed they may have proven that point many times over until they are convinced of their weakness.

You can learn to change. You can gain the power to turn off. Breakfast is the perfect meal with which to learn how. Especially if you eat the right kind of breakfast. Nighttime overeaters must practice eating breakfast for at least two weeks. It may take that long for your body to adjust to the change, but in the end, I think you will discover that it is much easier to limit the amount you eat at night when you are only moderately hungry than when you are famished.

Basic Breakfasts

I. Two slices whole wheat bread, plain or toasted, with one of the following:

> one ounce of your favorite hard cheese
> one-half cup low fat cottage cheese
> one scant tablespoon peanut butter
> one egg, soft-boiled or poached
> one glass low fat milk
> one cup of your favorite meat or vegetable soup

II. A serving of cereal that contains a large amount of whole grain, with a cup of low fat milk.

Do not use presweetened cereals and do not add sugar. Check the cereal box for size and calories per serving. If constipation on a diet has ever been a problem, try something like Bran Buds or 40 percent Bran Flakes. Or, add a small amount of bran to your regular cereal. Increase the amount slowly as necessary.

III. Optional with all breakfasts:
one serving of your favorite fruit or one-half cup fruit juice
coffee or tea (two cups a day, suggested upper limit)

The Nutritional Contents of a Good Breakfast

Breakfast, like all meals, should consist of foods that supply protein, fat, and carbohydrates. There should be some fat in all low calorie meals to help keep you satisfied and prevent hunger pangs. There should be some variety in all meals because the nutrients in food work together—if you eat just one food, you may miss obtaining nutrients that facilitate the utilization of other nutrients.

The fruit is optional at breakfast because some people feel uncomfortable with fruit first thing in the morning. Take it with you for a midmorning snack. You may also skip the fruit if it is on your luncheon or dinner menu.

Four servings of food in the grain category supply you with important amounts of fiber, B vitamins, iron, and a number of other minerals. With two slices of bread at breakfast, you will have eaten 50 percent of the grain foods (two of four servings) suggested by nutritionists in the Four Food Group Plan (chapter two).

Milk and dairy products (together with canned salmon and sardines) are your best sources for calcium—also, phosphorous and riboflavin, one of the B vitamins. With one serving at breakfast you get one of the two servings suggested in the Four Food Group Plan. If you prefer skim milk to low fat milk or cheese, that is all right, but I prefer some food with a small amount of fat in the morning. Fat is the last food component to leave the stomach during digestion. That is why it helps keep you satisfied longer than carbohydrates and somewhat longer than protein. Low fat milk may have about 30 calories more than skim milk per serving. It's a negligible price to pay for what may prove to be a considerable amount of satisfaction. It may save you from eating more later in the morning.

Each of the basic breakfasts totals between 200 and 300 calories, including the fruit. Figure 65 to 75 calories for each slice of bread, the egg, and a cup of most soups. Bouillion, however, has almost no calories—it's a free food. You can have all you want and eat more of something else. Most hard cheeses run about 100 calories an ounce, as does one-half cup of low fat cottage cheese. Peanut butter is about 100 calories a tablespoon and that's more than enough for two slices of bread.

If you have never measured or weighed food before, you will learn a lot by doing so. It only takes one time to get a clear picture of how large servings should be to supply a given number of calories. Therefore, measure the peanut butter or cottage cheese, and weigh the hard cheese. An inexpensive postal scale or small food scale works fine. Many overeaters underestimate their calories. You are only kidding yourself if you are one of them.

I like bread and cheese for breakfast best of all the recommendations. Cheese and peanut butter are a little higher in fat than the other selections, and I find that they keep most dieters satisfied for a longer period. If you have been accustomed to donuts or danish any time in the morning, or if you have any digestive discomfort or hunger pangs, be sure to try bread and cheese. Donuts and danish are far higher in calories from fat and sugar than that ounce of cheese, so the suggested breakfast, with a piece of fruit in reserve, not only provides more nutrients but also saves you calories in the long run.

Coffee and tea should be watched closely when you diet. I recommend that you try limiting yourself to a total of two cups a day, but I won't insist. Many successful dieters like to keep sipping all day, and use coffee or iced tea to good advantage. The problem arises when the stimulation of caffeine and other irritants in coffee combine with a decrease in food consumption. You may get a sour stomach or you may find yourself feeling nervous or physically jittery. Try sipping cold water plain or with a bit of lemon or lime juice, in place of the coffee or tea, or use herb teas (without caffeine) that you can find at health food stores or specialty food shops. You may note a great improvement in your general well-being, and much more comfortable digestive processes in as little as twenty-four hours.

DAY I

LUNCH
Large fruit salad
Optional: cheese, bread, or crackers

DINNER

Oven-baked chicken

Baked potato

Greens and sliced tomato, with choice of low calorie dressing, oil and vinegar, or real Italian dressing

Selection of herbs and seasoning: rosemary, parsley, basil, celery seed, and onion powder

Optional: milk, cheese, fruit

• *Lunch* •

USING FRUIT IN YOUR DIET

You can have certain fruits in unlimited quantities on this diet. *It means that you can use them as snacks as well as at main meals and never be hungry.* Fruit provides bulk to keep you regular, prevents the absorption of some fat calories, and is an excellent source of a wide variety of vitamins and minerals.

Eat at least two different fruits each day. Because of their low caloric density (few calories in relation to volume) you can eat all you want from the following list, day or night:

apples	pears	pineapple
oranges	melon	peaches
grapefruit	berries	

These fruits have approximately 60 calories in the average serving, and almost no one can eat them to excess because of their bulk. This makes them good substitutes for high calorie lunches, desserts, or snacks. Here is an example: A standard piece of apple pie that you might tack on to a meal as a dessert or possibly use as a snack in the evening before you go to bed, contains 300 to 350 calories. Try eating five or six medium-sized fresh apples or three or four whole grapefruit to equal that many calories—it's almost impossible. That's why fresh fruit from the list above can play such an important role, whether you are dieting or just trying to maintain your weight.

Fruits listed on the next page have a much greater caloric density than those you can eat in unlimited quantities. I suggest you use them to brighten up a salad, or plan on only one serving at a time. It is relatively easy to overeat on these. They have about 40 calories in the quantities listed here.

dates (2)   raisins (2 tablespoons)
dried prunes (2 large)   grapes or cherries (12 large)
figs (1)   apricots (2)
banana (1/2 small)

NUTS AND SEEDS

A tablespoon of seeds or chopped nuts (30–40 calories) can be added to a luncheon fruit salad. They provide an interesting contrast in flavor and texture. They also provide some protein and fat, two food components almost completely lacking in fruit. The protein and fat will make the fruit salad lunch stay with you for longer.

Sample Recipe

1 medium apple	2 dates
1 small pear	1 tablespoon sunflower seeds,
1 medium orange	chopped walnuts, or pecans
lemon juice	1 tablespoon shredded coconut

Cut apple and pear into bite-sized pieces. Place in two ounces of cold or iced water into which juice of one-half lemon or lime has been squeezed. You can use one teaspoon pure lemon juice in place of the fresh citrus fruit. This prevents discoloration and adds tartness. (You can squeeze lemon juice straight over the fruit, but I don't find that this strategy gives as good coverage as a mixture of cold water and juice.)

Add sectioned orange, cut to bite-size, and chopped or sliced dates (other dried fruit will also work very well).

Remove from lemon water to serving plate and sprinkle with coconut and sunflower seeds.

If you can eat it all (I doubt you can), you will have consumed about 300 calories. If not, save leftovers in the lemon water. The salad improves in flavor up to twenty–four hours.

You may want to get your second serving of a calcium-rich food at lunch. If so, add one-half cup low fat cottage cheese, a cup of yogurt, or an ounce of hard cheddar. All go very well with this particular salad. Or have a glass of milk as your beverage. If you have cheese or milk, save about one-third of the salad for a snack or for a dessert tonight.

Never be without a piece of fresh fruit at home or at work. It's your protection against the snack machine and gives you something to nibble on if you want to join your friends when they take a donut and coffee break. When they offer you that 200-calorie glazed donut you can say, "Thanks a lot, but I brought this apple for my snack today." You will be saving about 140 calories. If you do it daily, that's fourteen pounds of fat a year.

• *Dinner* •

CHICKEN

Chicken is an excellent low-calorie source of high quality protein. You will save many calories using chicken and fish as frequent substitutes for beef, pork, and lamb, although I will show you relatively low-calorie ways to prepare these meats as well.

Oven-baked is one of the best ways to prepare chicken. Always remove skin and fat before eating when trying to lose weight. Four ounces of oven-baked chicken has between 150 and 175 calories, whereas fried or roasted with skin has twice as much. Here are six quick ways to prepare flavor-rich oven-baked chicken.

1. Spread cut-up fryer on shallow, foil-lined baking pan. Sprinkle lightly with salt, pepper, and paprika. Bake on middle shelf for about one hour at 350°.

2. Sprinkle with garlic and/or onion powder.

3. Make a quick barbecue sauce with one part no-sugar soy sauce to two parts dry sherry. Let chicken marinate in sauce for two hours for fullest flavor, or spread sauce over the chicken as you bake it. Never use extra sweetener in your barbeque sauce.

4. Rub one or more herbs such as tarragon, chives, chervil, thyme, or parsley into the chicken before baking.

5. Add one or more of the above herbs to your barbecue sauce.

6. Make a mixture of soy sauce, ketchup, or chili sauce, garlic powder, and herbs. Add either a sprinkle of cayenne pepper, a dash of lemon juice, or a tablespoon of dry red wine. Spread liberally over chicken before baking.

No matter how you vary the proportions of ingredients for the variations I have just described, it is difficult to hurt chicken. As you experiment this week, you will soon get to know your taste preferences among the herbs and sauces I am suggesting. Part of the great joy of cooking comes when you feel free to discard your printed recipes. When you improvise each time you prepare a dish, it is different enough to be a pleasant surprise. It also speeds up the cooking process tremendously. You have tasty meals prepared in minutes.

POTATOES AND HERBS

A medium-sized baked potato (about two inches in diameter) has about 90 calories. Eaten with the skin, it has nutritional value similar to whole grain foods, plus some vitamin C. Potatoes can be a satisfying part of the diet once you learn to appreciate their flavor without drowning them in fat. Avoid french fries which have two to three times the number of calories as a baked potato.

To get acquainted with the flavor of a baked potato, as with all vegetables, it should be sampled plain and unadorned. A good baked potato is rather dry and flaky. Try a bite or two with nothing on it. Then try a pinch of salt on a bite-sized portion, next a bit of pepper, then a combination.

Some herbs that go well with potatoes are rosemary, basil, chives, in addition to the old standby—parsley. Go about your herb-and-potato tasting in this way: take a few leaves or sprigs of an herb and chew them up at the front of your mouth. Then roll the herb backwards to discover what part of your tongue is sensitive to that particular herb. Next, combine a bit of herb with a bit of potato— mashing it up well to release the flavor. Do it with each herb alone and then in combination. Let your family and friends do the experiment with you. Be prepared for people to respond differently to each herb. Sensitivity and taste preferences vary greatly. What is mild to you may be overpowering to someone else.

Many people come to prefer their baked potatoes absolutely plain, or with some salt and a few herbs. If you add butter and sour cream without caution, you can obtain two to three times more calories from the fat alone than is contained in the entire baked potato. You can, however, learn to use some fat if you like. Limit yourself to one pat (one teaspoon) of butter or two tablespoons of sour cream to a whole baked potato. They provide only thirty-five additional calories.

DINNER SALAD

Greens and sliced tomato with Low-cal, oil and vinegar, or Italian dressing make a fine salad. Mix up a bowl of spinach or collard greens, or try one or two varieties of lettuce. Greens have almost no calories and you can eat them freely. Slice up about one-half tomato for each person.

Forget your dietetic dressing for tonight. You can, if you prefer, use dietetic dressings in general, but if you tend to shy away from salad, it may be because of the way you prepare it. For tonight, it's okay to use your favorite dressing—the real stuff. I prefer oil and vinegar or an Italian for the following little experiment.

Most dieters don't know or haven't tried to learn how to use real dressings. It only takes one tablespoon (75 calories) to season a large salad for two people (e.g., half a head of lettuce) and, perhaps, one-and-a-half tablespoons to do four average servings, mixed in a large bowl. Keep a few leaves of your greens separate in order to be able to taste them plain, and then add the dressing. Mix well and let it stand for a few minutes to let the oil spread. Mix again.

At dinner, sample the lettuce plain, then the lettuce that has been mixed with some dressing. Then sprinkle some celery seed on a small portion, then onion powder, then both. I think you will be amazed at the variety of tastes you have created.

Now sample the tomato plain, then with celery seed and onion powder. The rosemary and basil that you used with the potato are also good with the tomato. Finish by mixing the tomato and lettuce salad together.

Playing with greens and tomatoes in this way, you have actually created several salads with several different tastes. This is the way to go about learning to create many simple dishes with flavors you may never have noticed before. As for calories, figure your share of the 75 that were in the dressing—perhaps 30, considering what stuck to the bowl. An entire medium-sized tomato has about 20. This salad provides a lot of satisfaction for under 75 calories.

In my opinion, very few dietetic dressings can give the satisfaction of the real thing. And as I have said before—that little bit of oil in the dressing makes the salad stay with you longer. I think you will also prefer the texture of salad when it has a small amount of oil. In the end, using a real dressing in small portions, you may eat more salad and not be tempted to eat the higher calorie foods that have far, far more fat in them than you have added to your salad.

Vegetables contain largely carbohydrates, but in very small quantities in comparison with their mass. As with fruits, their fiber makes fat pass through the system somewhat faster so that less may be absorbed. A leaf of lettuce has about 1 calorie; other greens have similar low values. A whole pound of greens raw has between 60 and 100 calories, compared with a pound of beef, which can have about 800 calories for the very leanest cut, well trimmed, to over 1500 for porterhouse and rib steaks. Greens are your best sources of vitamin A and many minerals. Use many different kinds.

As with the fruits I discussed at lunch, you can eat greens and other nonstarchy or low carbohydrate vegetables, such as celery and carrots, in unlimited quantities. Fall back on these foods for snacks.

SUMMING UP

So far your dinner has had:

chicken, 4 ozs.	175 calories	
potato, medium	90 calories (add 35 for 1 pat butter or 2 tbsp. sour cream)	
salad	75 calories	
Total	340 calories	

If you have stuck with the day's diet plan, you had about 600 calories before dinner, plus 340 now. Only 940 or so. Therefore, you have room for a second helping, or for milk, cheese, some more fruit, a slice of bread, or another potato. If you choose crackers to go with a piece of cheese for dessert, figure an average-size cracker at 15 to 20 calories. In general, crackers contain more fat than bread.

Daily Review

1. Write down everything you ate today and when.

2. Figure your estimated calories from the information I presented about the different foods.

3. Did you get two servings of a calcium-rich food?

4. Did you get plenty of fruits and vegetables?

5. Did you have any hunger pangs? If yes, did you have a fruit snack handy?

6. If you had more than two cups of coffee, did you experience any discomfort?

DAY II

LUNCH
Large vegetable salad
Optional: bread, cheese, fruit

DINNER
Beef steak or hamburger
Cooked vegetables
Optional: potato, bread, fruit, cheese

• *Lunch* •

INCREASE VEGETABLES IN YOUR DIET

All greens and vegetables in List 1 below can be used in unlimited quantities. They provide plenty of vitamins and minerals but very few calories. Vegetables high in vitamin A and vitamin C are marked as noted.

Vegetables in List 2 have thirty-five to forty calories per one-half cup serving. Active dieters can eat these in unlimited quantities as well. Because of their bulk, it is hard to overeat on any of them. They supply some protein in addition to carbohydrate, but virtually no fat.

List 3 contains relatively high calorie vegetables and legumes. Consider each serving of these as though you had eaten another slice of bread, since they have about sixty to ninety calories per half-cup portions cooked or in medium-sized pieces, except as noted.

List 1
Any amount may be eaten at each meal.

asparagus
bean sprouts
beans, green or wax
broccoli*†
cabbage (if raw†)
cauliflower
celery
chickory*

cucumber
eggplant
endive
escarole
greens, all kinds*
    (beet, chard, collard,
    kale, mustard, spinach,
    turnip)

(List continues on next page.)

lettuce	radish
mushrooms	romaine
okra	sauerkraut
parsley	summer squash
pepper, green*†	tomato†
pimento	zucchini

* Rich source of vitamin A.   † Rich source of vitamin C.

LIST 2

One serving equals ½ cup cooked vegetables or 1 cup raw vegetable.

artichoke	pumpkin*
beets	rutabaga
carrots*	squash
onions	(winter,* butternut, acorn)
peas, green	turnip

* Rich source of vitamin A

LIST 3

baked beans, no pork, ¼ cup	lima beans, fresh, cooked
	mixed vegetables
beans and peas, dried, cooked (black-eyed peas, kidney, lima, navy beans; split peas)	parsnips
	potato, white, 1 (two-inch diameter) baked or boiled
corn, sweet or white, ½ ear	potato, white, mashed
hominy	sweet potato or yam, ¼ cup

BASIC SALAD

Unlimited greens plus any vegetables of your choice from lists 1 and 2 above.

Dressings—one-half tablespoon of your favorite regular dressing, or vinegar, or lemon juice, or tomato juice blended with cottage cheese or yogurt plus a squeeze of lemon, or packaged low calorie dressing.

Herbs and seasonings—celery seed, onion powder, rosemary, basil, parsley. (See chart later in this chapter.)

Toppings—one ounce (four level tablespoons) grated cheese, or two heaping tablespoons chopped egg, a few croutons.

Cole slaw, or corn, pickle, tomato, or pepper relish, or three-bean salad can be used in moderation. The dressings and seasonings used in their preparation should be substituted for other dressings. Mix the slaw, relish, or three-bean salad with the rest of your salad.

FAST-FOOD SPECIAL SALAD

Many fast-food chains are now offering salad bars. Here is a typical nourishing salad which will have about one-half the calories of a hamburger, french fries, and a cola. Try it.

Spread grated carrots, chopped green peppers, and red cabbage to cover the bottom of your plate. Added chopped celery and sliced mushrooms. Place a few cherry tomatoes around the edges. Cover with some sprouts. All of these vegetables plus any greens can be used in unlimited quantities.

Add one-half cup cole slaw or three tablespoons relish or one ladle three-bean salad. Top with four tablespoons grated cheese (that's about an ounce).

No matter how many of the unlimited vegetables you put in a salad, you will find it hard to exceed 300 calories. The trick is in keeping the amount of fat down, but not eliminating it entirely. That little fat and protein provides the flavor that makes salads satisfying, day after day, and helps you last until your next meal.

• *Dinner* •

BEEF

Beef is an excellent source of protein, B vitamins, and minerals such as iron and phosphorous. Unfortunately, in most cuts of beef, you obtain more fat calories than you do protein. That is why if you get your protein from meat, a high protein diet turns out to be a high fat diet. In a top grade porterhouse steak, nearly 80 percent of the caloric content is from fat. Regular hamburger is almost as high. Therefore, you must choose the leanest cuts of steak and ground beef that you can find. Trim all extra fat. An eight-ounce strip of rib eye well trimmed will end up weighing five–six ounces cooked and supply 300 to 350 calories. So will lean hamburger, provided you press out any extra fat either in the pan or on paper towels after cooking. You will save 100 to 200 calories on medium rare hamburgers if you press and drain them well.

For pan- or oven-broiled beef, sprinkle with a small amount of salt, pepper, and other seasonings of your choice. You need no extra fat for cooking.

Teriyaki: One tablespoon no-sugar soy sauce (per steak), dash worchestershire, ½ teaspoon ginger (per steak), garlic powder, pepper. Mix together in a dish large enough to hold meat. Turn in sauce so that both sides are covered. If you choose a tough cut of meat, puncture with tines of a fork so sauce can penetrate. Let stand a few minutes for tender cuts, and from one-half hour up to several hours for cuts less tender. Just before the steaks are finished cooking, pour the remains of the marinade over them and heat. After you remove the steak from the pan, you can add a small amount of water or dry red table wine and make a tasty sauce. It's excellent over vegetables or over baked potato.

For flank steak, prepare twice the amount of marinade and add minced scallions. Refrigerate steak in marinade overnight in a plastic bag. Broil and slice thinly for a low fat, tender treat—one of my favorite low calorie cuts.

Teriyaki with mushrooms: Broil, then top steak with mushrooms a few minutes before steaks are done. If pan broiling, lightly grease the pan with a small amount of fat from the meat. Half-cook the mushrooms, covered, on low heat. You can add a tablespoon of the teriyaki sauce to create a bit of steam and to speed the process. Place mushrooms to the side, with any remaining liquid from the pan, and cook steaks. Return mushrooms to the pan for the final two minutes of cooking.

Flamed with brandy: Pan broil. Just before the steaks are finished, turn the heat up to high, add one ounce of brandy, and flame. The meat will be somewhat sweeter than normal. Flamed teriyaki with mushrooms is a special treat.

Hamburgers can be cooked exactly as pan-broiled steak. You have never tasted one this good.

COOKED VEGETABLES

Try one of the following three suggestions:

1. Sliced onions with greens, green beans, or summer squash

2. Steamed broccoli, summer squash, and cabbage
3. Mushrooms with spinach or green beans

HERB AND VEGETABLE COMBINATIONS

Parsley goes with almost all vegetables
Tarragon with cabbage, celery
Bay leaf, minced onion, and a squeeze of lemon with asparagus
Basil, onion, and garlic powder with green beans
Rosemary with lima beans or carrots
Oregano and basil with eggplant
Potatoes with rosemary, marjoram, dill, or basil
Tomatoes with rosemary, oregano, and basil

QUICK CREAM SAUCE FOR VEGETABLES

For four servings, add one can cream of onion, celery, mushroom, chicken, or tomato soup without extra water. A 10½ ounce can of a cream soup will add 50 to 75 calories to each serving. Limit yourself to a single helping prepared in this way while dieting.

SUMMING UP

A bread and cheese breakfast, a piece of fruit, and a large luncheon salad add up to approximately 600 calories. Your beef dinner contained around 350. If you had a baked potato (90 calories), you can finish up with some fruit and another piece of cheese or some milk. Without the baked potato there is room for bread or crackers with cheese and some fruit for dessert.

Daily Review

1. Write down everything you ate today and when.
2. Figure your estimated calories from the information I presented about the different foods.
3. Did you get two servings of a calcium-rich food?
4. Did you get plenty of fruits and vegetables?
5. Did you have any hunger pangs? If yes, did you have a fruit snack handy?
6. If you had more than two cups of coffee, did you experience any discomfort?

DAY III

LUNCH

Sandwich, two slices whole grain bread, two slices any combination cheese, sliced ham, turkey, chicken, or lean beef. Ketchup, mustard, or one teaspoon mayonnaise as spread.

Lettuce, tomato, sprouts, or other vegetables in unlimited quantities.

Optional: fruit, milk products, meat or vegetable soup

DINNER

Skillet-fried vegetables with one half cup brown rice, or baked potato, or two slices of toast

Four tablespoons grated cheese

Fruit

• *Lunch* •

MAKING A NUTRITIOUS LOW CALORIE SANDWICH

Two slices whole grain bread, cheese and/or meat, and some lettuce and tomato or other vegetables supply a nutritious, well-rounded lunch. The sandwich prepared in this way contains protein, carbohydrate, and fat, and a wide range of other essential nutrients. Use only real sliced ham, turkey, or beef and not processed meats such as bologna or salami which are especially high in fat and added salt. You can use one teaspoon of mayonnaise (35 calories) or all the ketchup or mustard you like. This is a good time to learn just how little mayonnaise it takes to season a sandwich well, provided you also add some lettuce and tomato or other vegetables such as sprouts.

A sandwich of this size with mayonnaise will contain about 300 calories, just like your fruit and vegetable salads.

It is not necessary to shy away from bread on a diet. As you recall, four servings of grain products are recommended in the Four Group Plan. On days on which you are having less meat, such as today, it is a good time to add more bread since many of the same vitamins and minerals that you find in meat are also found in whole grains. In fact, it is possible to design a healthy low calorie diet with very little meat and six to eight slices of whole grain bread daily.

You can finish off with fruit if you are still hungry, since an active dieter can eat all the fruit and vegetables he or she wants. However, if you choose a cream or vegetable soup for lunch, you will be getting between sixty to seventy five calories per cup. In that case, I would save fruit or vegetables for a mid-afternoon snack.

• *Dinner* •
SKILLET-FRIED VEGETABLES WITH BROWN RICE

Skillet frying is a variation of stir frying that can be done without special equipment. Any saucepan, large frying pan, or skillet will work.

If you are already experienced in stir frying, do it your way.

Here is my quick recipe (thirty minutes from start to finish) using any old large sauce pan or deep skillet with a cover.

1 green pepper	cabbage
2 medium onions	green (spinach or collards pre-
2–4 cloves garlic	ferred)
4–6 stalks celery	1 tablespoon no-sugar soy sauce
4 large carrots	fresh ground pepper

Start rice or potatoes one hour before serving. Cook one cup of rice in two cups of water. As part of the liquid, use vegetable or meat stock, or add two bouillon cubes to the water.

Melt one tablespoon of butter or warm one tablespoon of oil in your skillet as you begin to slice your vegetables. Over medium-low heat, add the sliced green pepper, followed by carrots in one-half-inch pieces, followed by sliced onions, chopped garlic, and celery in two-inch pieces. Cover and reduce heat to low. Wash your greens and add in the order you like cooked longest. Cabbage goes in before the greens, which take only a few minutes. Serve your vegetables while they are still crisp. Just before removing from the pan, add one to two tablespoons of no-sugar soy sauce and season with ground pepper and herbs of your choice. Marjoram, thyme, and celery seed are excellent. Serves four.

Expect to get about the same amount of salty flavor from one tablespoon of soy sauce that you get from one-half teaspoon of salt. These quantities have about equivalent amounts of sodium (one gram). I think you will find that one to two tablespoons of soy sauce is enough for the entire serving for four.

Considering how few calories there are in your vegetables, and how little fat per serving, it is very difficult to go over 300 calories with a heaping serving of your skillet-fry on one-half cup cooked brown rice (90 calories) topped with four tablespoons grated cheese (100 calories). For variation, try this skillet fry over toast or a baked potato.

Vegetables served with cheese and a whole grain such as brown rice are a particularly good substitute for a meat dish since the combination of vegetables, grain, and cheese enhances the quality of protein available from any single food eaten separately. When you are eating a reduced amount of meat on a given day, increase your grains, vegetables, and cheese in order to obtain adequate protein and B vitamins.

SUMMING UP

With this low calorie dinner, you have had about 900 calories so far today. This means you can have another portion of the stir fry or a slice of bread and an ounce of cheese for dessert with fruit. Cheese can count either as a calcium rich food or as a protein (meat) food in the Four Food Group Plan. For example, count your first two servings of cheese in the calcium category, and the third in the meat group.

Looking at your fat calories, you may have had as many as 70 from added calories in the butter or oil, and mayonnaise. You may have as many as 240 calories hidden in the cheese, the meat in your luncheon sandwich, or peanut butter. When you add those calories together you will see that in today's diet you had just about 25 percent of your total calories in fat.

The high fat foods in your diet, which you are eating in very limited quantities, are peanut butter, hard cheese, mayonnaise, butter or oil, and salad dressings. Over 70 percent of the calories in these foods comes from fat, and in the case of mayonnaise, butter, margarine, or oil, 100 percent of the calories is fat. Using fat or oil judiciously, according to the Seven-Day Plan, however, you are not likely to take in more than 200 calories from these foods in any given day.

Fish, fowl, and lean meat, as well as low fat milk, have 20 to 30 percent of their caloric content in fat. Virtually all of your grains, vegetables, and fruits are fat free.

By limiting your servings in the high fat (70 to 100 percent) food categories to two or no more than three per day, you will have no trouble keeping your fat calories at approximately 25 percent of your total daily intake.

Daily Review

1. Write down everything you ate today and when.

2. Figure your estimated calories from the information I presented about the different foods.

3. Did you get two servings of a calcium-rich food?

4. Did you get plenty of fruits and vegetables?

5. Did you have any hunger pangs? If yes, did you have a fruit snack handy?

6. If you had more than two cups of coffee, did you experience any discomfort?

DAY IV

LUNCH

Spinach salad with sliced mushrooms, green pepper, and chopped egg

Sliced Bermuda onion optional

One-half tablespoon regular dressing or low calorie dressing to taste

One slice whole wheat bread or six crackers

Fruit and cheese (or other milk products)

DINNER

Fish, baked, broiled, or poached

Your choice of cooked vegetables

Fruit

• *Lunch* •

A spinach salad prepared as suggested tends to go well with oil and vinegar or Italian dressing. Mix the vegetables with one-half tablespoon regular dressing per serving and let sit a few minutes. Then toss again to let the dressing blend. Including a chopped egg, the dressing, and the bread, it is hard to eat more than 200 calories worth of this salad.

For variety, try a spinach salad with two tablespoons fresh grated parmesan cheese in place of the egg, or some herb bread crumbs tossed with the salad dressing.

Finish the meal with a piece of fruit and a serving of some milk product to be sure you are getting your calcium for the day.

• *Dinner* •

FISH

Fish are excellent sources of high grade protein and a wide variety of minerals. Fish are categorized as fresh water, salt water, or shell fish. Each type differs somewhat from the other in nutritional value. Therefore, it is a good idea to vary the kind of fish you eat. Fish have very little fat and those that have somewhat more, such as halibut, mackerel, and salmon are good sources of vitamins A and D. However, the more fatty fish generally contain no more than 30 percent fat calories.

The following fish are excellent broiled: fillets of turbot, flounder, and sole; salmon and swordfish steaks; small rainbow trout, one-half to three-quarters pound.

> Brush fish lightly with oil, or pour a small amount of oil in a shallow foil lined baking dish or broiler pan. Sprinkle salt and pepper on the oil and swish the fish around on both sides. You're ready. Broil on the second shelf down from the top of your oven. Turn your fish over to brown on both sides for a total cooking time of between 12 to 14 minutes for fillets, a little longer for the whole small rainbow trout.

> *A lemon herb butter sauce* poured over broiled fish is delicious.

> In a saucepan over low heat, melt one tablespoon butter for every two servings of fish. Add the juice of half a lemon, a teaspoon of chives, and a half teaspoon parsley or chervil. Warm, but do not brown. Spoon a portion over each fish or fish fillet as it is served. For an *almond butter sauce* you can add chopped or ground almonds to the lemon butter instead of the herbs.

Fillets and fish steaks do well baked in a covered baking dish or wrapped and sealed in aluminum foil. The following bouillon goes well with all varieties of fish and is especially delicious for salmon steaks or a whole salmon baked in foil:

one-half cup white wine
one slice lemon
a small onion chopped
Simmer 15 to 30 minutes.

your favorite herbs
(try ½ teasp. thyme, basil,
rosemary, and tarragon)

Place fish in baking dish or foil. Add salt and pepper. Pour the bouillon over the fish. Cover and bake in the oven at 375° about twenty minutes for fillets or fifteen minutes a pound for whole fish.

You can be very creative with sauces and bouillons. Fifty/fifty white wine and water with a little salt and pepper and minced onion is a perfectly acceptable bouillon for baking. Or, try a can of minced clams and a few slices of tomato with salt and pepper. An unbelievably easy fish parmesan is prepared by simply covering your favorite fish fillets with a can of Italian tomato sauce and sprinkling it with parmesan cheese. Bake this one uncovered in the oven at 400° for about twenty minutes until the cheese begins to brown.

Figure six ounces of fish or a whole rainbow trout at around 300 calories. The lemon-herb butter contains around 20 calories a teaspoonful.

VEGETABLES

Choose your favorites, or try one of these three suggestions. They go well with fish.

French beans with sliced mushrooms. Steam or boil in one-quarter cup water. Salt and pepper to taste and add one teaspoon of butter for the pot if you like a little fat flavor. Additional seasonings include garlic or onion powder, basil, chervil, and parsley. This will contain approximately 40 calories per serving.

Lima beans. Cook in ¼ cup water. Add two teaspoons of butter and one-half teaspoon rosemary for two cups hot beans. Contains about 90 calories for a half cup. Remember that lima beans serve as an extra bread selection, just as do potatoes and corn.

Sliced onions and green peas. A large sliced white onion with sixteen ounces of peas cooked in ¼ cup water. Start the onion first, and when translucent, add the peas and cook for about six more minutes. Add, if you like, one teaspoon of butter for the pot, although this particular combination is delicious without any fat. Basil is an excellent seasoning for onions and green peas. Contains approximately 30 calories per half-cup serving.

This has been an extremely low calorie day because of the low fat content in your spinach salad and in the fish. Figure the calories yourself. Think for a moment to determine whether you have had two milk servings and if not, finish off the evening meal with some fruit and cheese or a glass of milk.

Daily Review

1. Write down everything you ate today and when.

2. Figure your estimated calories from the information I presented about the different foods.

3. Did you get two servings of a calcium food?

4. Did you get plenty of fruits and vegetables?

5. Did you have any hunger pangs? If yes, did you have a fruit snack handy?

6. If you had more than two cups of coffee, did you experience any discomfort?

DAY V

LUNCH

Choice of cottage cheese, tuna, or salmon salad with assorted fresh
    vegetables
Slice whole wheat bread or crackers

DINNER

Herbed pork (or lamb)
Baked potato
Cooked vegetables
Optional: Fruit, cheese

• Lunch •

The salad today is a typical dieter's special and one of the better ones that you can find in most restaurants as well as one that you can prepare at home. This particular salad, regardless of which protein food you use, has a good balance of all the essential nutrients—protein, carbohydrate and fat, as well as variety of vitamins and minerals. The cottage cheese can count as a serving in the meat or milk group of the Four Food Group Plan. Tuna and salmon are low calorie, high protein fish, but only the salmon is high in calcium because it contains the bones of the fish. If you wish, you can substitute five medium sardines which are also rich in calcium, for the salmon. Stuffed in a tomato, with lettuce and a few other fresh vegetables, such as a couple of carrot sticks, celery, or radishes, this sardine salad provides plenty of vitamins A and C. These are the two vitamins provided primarily by vegetables and fruits.

An entire 6½ ounce can of tuna fish in spring water has only 200 calories. And salmon has about the same amount if you choose Chum or Pink. The more expensive sockeye variety has much more fat and is considerably more caloric. Five medium-sized sardines contain about 120 calories. Low fat cottage cheese will have between 80 and 110 calories per half cup. You have to check labels to be sure since brands vary.

Because your vegetables and protein dish are so low in calories, you can use up to one whole tablespoon of regular salad dressing, but I doubt you will need that much for the usual-size salad. You can, of course, use your favorite low calorie dressing since there is enough fat in the cottage cheese, tuna, or salmon to make this a satisfying meal with staying power. Caloric content can range from about 175 calories for cottage cheese on tomato with vegetables, no salad dressing to about 300 if you choose the salmon and use a full tablespoon of mayonnaise, which, in itself contains 100 calories. As you become more sensitive to flavor, one teaspoon of salad dressing may prove to be enough, especially if you use a squeeze of lemon juice which enhances the flavor of the tuna, salmon, and sardines.

This is an excellent luncheon dish to order in most restaurants since they tend to use the low fat varieties of fish. They are cheaper.

• *Dinner* •

Pork is a high quality protein dish and may be your best bargain in meats. You obtain nutrition approximately equal to beef or lamb at a fraction of the price. Many cuts of pork are very fatty, however, so you must use care in selection and preparation.

Pork and other meats are a primary source of B vitamins, particularly thiamin, and a relatively good source of iron. People on reduced caloric intakes are often deficient in these nutrients, especially iron. When we are low in B vitamins or iron, we are low in energy and easily fatigued because B vitamins are essential to the breakdown of carbohydrates to glucose and then the utilization of glucose for energy. All of this metabolic activity requires the presence of oxygen, which in turn depends upon an adequate supply of iron. Iron is responsible for the ability of both hemoglobin and myoglobin to transport oxygen (and carbon dioxide, a waste product of metabolism) in the blood. Even if you have an adequate supply of glucose in your body, you cannot use it efficiently when you are low in iron.

PREPARATION

This recipe for herbed pork is one of my favorites and I love to prepare it for my friends. Practice with it once, and then you may want to show it off, too.

Choose lean loin or rib chops, or tenderloin cutlets, cut 1 to 1½ inches thick. Trim off excess fat. The chops are likely to be somewhat tough, so coat them lightly with a small smount of soy sauce, puncture with a fork, and let them marinate before cooking for at least two hours (better twenty-four). This procedure is not necessary for tenderloin. Mix about one-half teaspoon each of a variety of herbs—I prefer rosemary, thyme, tarragon, oregano, sage, and basil—with pepper and garlic powder to taste, for four large chops. Rub the mixture well into the meat. Place in skillet with one-half cup water, and very gently simmer, covered, for 45 minutes. Do not boil; it makes the meat tough. Remove chops in order to pour off and save any remaining liquid. If you have trimmed the meat well, there will be almost no fat on top of the liquid. You can remove the fat, but leave all the herbs.

Return chops to the pan and brown on both sides. When done, place them on a warm platter. Return liquid to pan for warming since it makes a delicious sauce. Taste and add more water as necessary, or a quarter cup dry white table wine if you prefer. Simmer and keep tasting since the flavor changes quickly and drastically as the liquid evaporates. Don't worry about the calories in these juices. You have trimmed the fat and the alcohol in wine evaporates, leaving only a few sugar calories. This sauce takes about two minutes to make, but if your chops have cooled too much, you can return them to the pan for a minute just before serving.

Serve juices on the chops, baked potato or vegetables.

Loin and rib lamb chops can be herbed in the same way as pork. Three small ribs, 1 to 1½ inches thick make a serving. Pan broil (no water) uncovered until done (fifteen minutes for medium rare). Remove chops and add one-half cup water or dry red table wine to make your sauce. Simmer and taste until the flavor is just right.

A six-ounce portion of lean pork or lamb, will contain about 400 calories.

VEGETABLES

A good crunchy combination of steamed vegetables to go with pork or lamb includes broccoli or cauliflower, plus celery, carrots, and onions.

SUMMING UP

Figure your calories. Even after this hearty dinner you have room for a piece of fruit as a dessert or bedtime snack.

Daily Review

1. Write down everything you ate today and when.

2. Figure your estimated calories from the information I presented about the different foods.

3. Did you get two servings of a calcium-rich food?

4. Did you get plenty of fruits and vegetables?

5. Did you have any hunger pangs? If yes, did you have a fruit snack handy?

6. If you had more than two cups of coffee, did you experience any discomfort?

DAY VI

LUNCH

Dieter's special: ground beef patty, cottage cheese, fruit, or lettuce and tomato, one slice whole wheat bread

DINNER

Macaroni and peas with tarragon butter, salad, fruit

• *Lunch* •

THE DIETER'S SPECIAL

Without care, the dieter's special can turn out to be a high calorie bomb. An eight-ounce (raw weight), restaurant-grade hamburger may contain close to 500 calories, whereas prepared at home from ground extra lean beef, it will contain around 300. You must press out all of the fat from regular restaurant-grade hamburgers to save those 200 calories. Creamed cottage cheese can have as much as 140 calories per half cup versus 80 for low fat. Each piece of canned fruit in heavy syrup can contain about 20 calories more than the water packed or fresh variety. This dieter's special, with a large eight-ounce burger, can vary from as little as 400 to around 700 calories.

If you order the dieter's special in a restaurant, inquire about the size of the hamburger and the kind of cottage cheese. Before eating the hamburger, press out all the fat (I have gotten two full tablespoons of fat squeezed from a cooked eight-ounce dieter's special). Choose a four-ounce hamburger size if they have it. If the cottage cheese is regular creamed, eat about one-quarter cup. Choose lettuce and tomato over canned fruit.

If you press the fat from a four-ounce hamburger, you can reduce its caloric content to around 150. Eat only one-quarter cup creamed cottage cheese (one-half cup low fat) and, with lettuce and tomato, you still have room for a slice of bread or a half dozen crackers before you reach that nice round 300-calorie number for your lunch. That's a far cry from the 700-calorie potential in the dieter's special. The nutritional quality is excellent—you have a meat serving, a milk serving, one-half of two vegetable servings (assuming small portions of lettuce and tomato), and a grain. Not bad for 300 calories.

• *Dinner* •

PASTA AND PASTA DISHES

Whereas dieters may often mistakenly believe they are eating a low calorie plate when they order the dieter's special on today's luncheon menu, they just as often mistakenly believe that pasta dishes must be highly caloric. As I will show you, it all depends upon the fat content. A cup of spaghetti with a fatty meat sauce can easily contain 400 calories—but 1½ cups of tonight's main pasta course has only 225.

Using whole wheat pasta you obtain the nutritional value of the whole grain at a low cost and few calories (See table 2 in this chapter). By mixing pasta with one or more vegetables and adding meat, fish, or cheese in small quantities, you enhance the nutritional value of each food. As I mentioned earlier, nutrients work together. The protein in a milk, fish, or meat product enhances the value of the protein in vegetables and grains. The interactive facilitation of vitamins and minerals, while too complex to be fully discussed in a book of this nature, works in a similar way. For example, calcium, vitamins D and C, and iron all work together. The B vitamins need each other. The body requires some of each of a variety of nutrients if it is to make full use of any one. In some cases, the food elements must be eaten at the same time for best utilization. This is particularly true of nutrients not stored to any large extent in the body, such as vitamin C, many B vitamins, and the protein we obtain from animal and plant sources. They are best eaten along with the other nutrients with which they interact.

You don't need to be an expert in nutrition, however, to eat in a nutritious way. Through the ages, combination food dishes have evolved naturally to meet the body's needs—beans and rice, spaghetti and tomato sauce with meat or cheese, pasta or other grains with vegetables, plus a little cheese or meat product. Just eat a wide variety of foods, combine them in any way that appeals to you and keep the fat and sugar to a minimum.

Here is a recipe for preparing pasta:

12 ozs. whole wheat macaroni
8 oz. package of snow peas (or regular green peas)
1 6½ oz. can of crab meat (or tuna or boned chicken)

salt, fresh ground pepper
2 cloves garlic minced
1 small onion minced
1 tablespoon butter or oil
½ teaspoon tarragon

Saute garlic and onion with butter in large skillet over low heat until translucent. Cook macaroni in large amount of water for ten minutes; add snow peas and cook two to four minutes more after pot returns to a boil. If you are using regular green peas, add to pot at eight minutes and cook for six minutes longer. Drain. Add to skillet with crab meat and tarragon. Salt and pepper to taste. Warm for two to four minutes. Serves four.

One and one-half cups of this pasta contain approximately 225 calories.

SALAD

Greens or spinach with your favorite dressing.

SUMMING UP

By now you can see that all the meal plans leave room for fruit as a dessert or snack. Tonight's meal contains around 300 calories, lunch contained 300, and breakfast between 200 and 300. Thus, you can use fruit or the low calorie vegetables at any time of the day or night. The milk food category, however, is likely to be slighted in many low calorie diets. Check your day to see whether you have gotten that second serving of a milk product. If not, have a piece of cheese with that fruit, or a glass of low fat milk. As you become more active, your calcium requirements may increase slightly, since the increase in activity is causing your bones to get harder and stronger.

Daily Review

1. Write down everything you ate today and when.

2. Figure your estimated calories from the information I presented about the different foods.

3. Did you get two servings of a calcium-rich food?

4. Did you get plenty of fruits and vegetables?

5. Did you have any hunger pangs? If yes, did you have a fruit snack handy?

6. If you had more than two cups of coffee, did you experience any discomfort?

DAY VII

LUNCH
Fruit salad, or lunch of your choice

DINNER
Pot roast of beef with tomato sauce and vegetables
Optional: greens, fruit, cheese

• *Lunch* •

It's time to start some of your own planning. I suggest a fruit salad because it is a good one to have more than once a week. This time try different fruits and nuts. But there is no need to follow that recommendation. You have now experimented with six different luncheon menus, each around 300 calories. Survey your day's menus to see what you have missed at breakfast and what's coming up for tonight and plan accordingly. Most people in this country eat an abundance of protein foods, so as long as you are getting plenty of fruits and vegetables, and starting the day with whole grain bread or cereal, the only nutritional components you may miss are those in the milk group. If you are not a milk drinker, you may have to go out of your way to get adequate calcium.

• *Dinner* •

Pot roast of beef, with tomato sauce and vegetables—here is your legendary total meal in one pot. Easy to prepare and as with all combination meat and vegetable dishes, it supplies a wide variety of nutrients.

Choose your meat carefully because your leanest cuts—flank and lean round steak—have only a fraction of the calories in chuck or rump roast. These last are delicious, of course, but not necessarily cheaper after you cut away all excess fat. And no matter how much you trim, there is much more fat running through the meat, so, you will have a lot of skimming to do after the roast is done.

I suggest you make an extra large recipe because this roast improves for several days, and any leftover sauce can be used with pasta.

4 lbs. bone-in roast or 2 lbs. flank steak	bay leaf
	Italian seasonings
2–4 cloves garlic, minced or crushed	1 28-oz. can peeled tomatoes
	1 15-oz. tomato sauce or puree
2 medium onions	¾ cup hearty red table wine
1 green pepper	2 tbsp. no-sugar soy sauce
4–5 stalks celery	dash worcestershire
6 large carrots	fresh ground pepper
4–6 medium potatoes	

Place meat with garlic in large roasting pan (no need to brown). Spread thinly sliced onion and green pepper around and on top. Add large pieces of celery, carrots, and potatoes—quartered is recommended because you don't want them to dissolve and disappear in the sauce.

Pour tomatoes and tomato sauce over the meat and vegetables, mix up the soy, worcestershire, and wine and add to pot, together with bay leaf, Italian seasonings, and fresh ground pepper. Commercial Italian seasonings are available, or make your own from oregano, marjoram, rosemary, basil, sage, thyme, and tarragon. If you don't like to mix so many flavors, try just oregano and basil together, or marjoram and thyme. By now you should have a good idea how these will affect your food.

Cook in 250° oven for four to five hours for greatest flavor. Mix the tomato sauce and vegetables two or three times during the cooking. Taste the sauce about an hour before serving—it may require more salt.

The roast can be cooked faster, at 325° for three to four hours, but the flavor won't be full until tomorrow if you do that. Do not serve until the meat falls apart when you prod it with a fork. Let it roast on low heat until it is very tender. Skim the fat. Approximately eight servings.

SALAD

You already have your meal in the pot tonight, but a green salad with oil and vinegar or Italian dressing gives you an interesting contrast in flavor and texture.

SUMMING UP

With a four ounce, all-lean meat portion, plus a whole potato, with plenty of sauce and other vegetables, it will be hard to exceed 450 calories unless you have failed to remove the fat. Under those conditions, your calorie count can easily double.

This dinner, combined with a 300-calorie breakfast, and a 300-calorie lunch still leaves you room for that fruit snack or that milk product if you haven't had your two servings today.

Daily Review

1. Write down everything you ate today and when.
2. Figure your estimated calories from the information I presented about the different foods.
3. Did you get two servings of a calcium-rich food?

4. Did you get plenty of fruits and vegetables?

5. Did you have any hunger pangs? If yes, did you have a fruit snack handy?

6. If you had more than two cups of coffee, did you experience any discomfort?

Principles of the Double Your Fat Loss Diet

I. *Low fat*   But not *no* fat. Small amounts keep you satisfied and add flavor. No fried food.

II. *High carbohydrate*   Plenty of fruits and vegetables, but no sweets or processed snack foods.

III. *A small breakfast*   Keeps your energy level up and prevents that uncontrollable night-time eating drive.

IV. *A wide variety of foods*   Insures adequate nutrition as well as the avoidance of a concentration of any food additives or pesticides that might accompany overconsumption of a single food.

V. *Several different foods at each meal*   Especially lunch and dinner. Facilitates adequate absorption of all nutrients.

Construct Your Own Plan

1. *Breakfast.* Follow the outline at the beginning of the chapter. Total: 200–300 calories.

2. *Lunch.* Use any one of the six lunches in my Seven-Day Plan as often as you like. Or make your own with fruits, vegetables, a grain serving, and a small portion of lean meat, fish, fowl, cheese, or milk products. Add only a small amount of fat—one teaspoon of mayonnaise for a sandwich, one-half tablespoon of salad dressing for a salad. A small amount of fat will keep you satisfied for longer periods. Total: about 300 calories.

3. *Dinner.* A larger meat, fish, or fowl serving with vegetables and either a grain or potato. For variety, use low fat pasta dishes with vegetables and a little meat, fowl, or fish. Learn to use seasonings for variety and flavor. Total: about 450 calories.

The day's total of 950–1050 calories leaves you room for fruit and cheese desserts, or other milk products, or a bedtime snack. Do not eat less than 1200 calories.

4. *Don't be compulsive about the calorie count.* Don't suffer when

you are hungry. Use fresh fruits and vegetables freely so that you are not tempted to revert to high-fat foods or rich desserts. If you splurge on fruits or vegetables, you will rarely go more than 100 or so calories over 1200. You will still lose weight at about a pound a week if you add as many as two fruit snacks during the day, and two more to allay any hunger at night.

Think ahead—you *will* be able to eat high calorie foods once you reach desirable weight *provided you have become active*. Right now, you can't eat high calorie foods that have little other nutritional value outside of their calories and lose weight efficiently.

Rules for Preparing All Recipes the Low Calorie Way

You can prepare all of your own favorite recipes and save many calories by simply reducing the fat and added sugar components to a minimum. First, try halving the amounts called for, and, depending on the outcome, halve again the next time.

You never need more than one tablespoon of fat for sautéing onions, peppers, and garlic before combining with other ingredients. Cover the skillet, do it on medium heat or lower, and possibly add a bit of water. Many times, simmering in water without any fat will prove satisfactory.

For stuffings, sauces, and gravies, try water, dry wine, or vegetable or meat bouillon, in place of butter and cream. For example, many rich stuffings for fish and fowl call for as much as a quarter cup of butter and a quarter cup of heavy cream, which contain a total of about 600 calories. I find that these recipes are just as good if I use no more than one tablespoon of butter for flavor and a fifty-fifty mixture of water and white wine, or bouillon and wine, which will contain between 100 and 150 calories. Sometimes you can substitute low fat milk for cream (12 calories per ounce instead of 100).

When making meat sauces for pasta and casseroles, always be sure to cook the ground beef in such a way as to be able to press the meat and pour off the fat before combining with the other ingredients. This can save you 200 to 400 calories a pound.

At the end of this chapter, I present an assortment of delicious low fat, low sugar recipes. You can use them on my Seven-Day Plan as substitutes, and over and over again whether you are dieting or not. Examine the style of cooking in these recipes and then create your own culinary originals.

Eating Out on the Seven-Day Plan

There is no problem eating out on the Seven-Day Plan. Most restaurants will have one or another of the lunches I suggest. As for dinner, here are some pointers that you can use in selecting any restaurant meal.

I. Choose clear soups, fowl, or lean meats, or fish broiled either without butter or just brushed lightly if you can trust the chef. If the fish proves to be on the dry side, just one-half pat of butter (one-half teaspoon) will supply all the fat you need for flavor and texture. You can spread it at the table yourself and add a squeeze of lemon.

II. Order any sandwich or salad with dressing on the side. Use diet dressings, or as I prefer, no more than one-half tablespoon of the genuine article. Use mustard freely and ketchup with moderation. A tablespoon of ketchup contains 16 calories, a good part of which is supplied by sugar.

III. Avoid creamed soups, breaded or fried meats, french fried potatoes, potato chips, milk shakes, and desserts. Choose sliced chicken, ham, or beef instead of processed meats. Avoid soft drinks. All 160 calories in a twelve-ounce soft drink, *or about 10 teaspoons full,* are sugar calories.

IV. Think in terms of 300 calories for lunch and about 600 for dinner. After studying and using the Seven-Day Plan just once, you will have a good idea of what foods to include to reach these totals.

V. You are always perfectly safe at lunch times *if you carry your own fruit.* If there is nothing at all on the menu that fits your plan, you can order toast and a slice of cheese, or a side-order (four-ounce) meat patty, and a cup of tea or coffee. An apple, pear, or an orange in your pocket, bag, or purse is a symbol of your resolve to stick with your plan. Just order something simple to go with it.

Find the restaurants that serve the food you want and get on friendly terms with the owners, the cooks, and the people who will be serving you. If your favorite establishments are very busy during the times you usually eat, make a point to eat one meal during off hours. At that time, explain to the person who usually serves you what you are trying to do and ask for someone to tell you how the dishes on the menu are prepared. This can turn out to be both fun and informative. Then see if the restaurant will cook their usual dishes the way you want in the future, that is, with very little or no fat.

Because so many overweight people feel they cannot eat out and still conserve calories, and because they feel uncomfortable about asking for special consideration in food preparation, I decided to find out just what difficulties people will face if they do as I suggest. I visited every kind of restaurant, from coffee shops to the most exclusive and expensive establishments during my travels in every one of the continental United States. I would explain that I had to follow a special diet—very little fat and sugar. I would ask how each dish was prepared and find out if the restaurant would prepare things the way I wanted. I was pleasantly surprised at the collaboration I received at all times. In many cases, if the owner were not busy, he or she would come to chat with me about food preparation. They often would tell me the calorie content of their dishes and I learned many new recipes.

I also discovered an invaluable piece of information for dieters. On hundreds of occasions, at restaurants that showed no fruit on their menus, I would ask my waiter or waitress at the end of my meal if there was any fresh fruit available in the kitchen—an apple or an orange if nothing else. Except for certain chains of fast food restaurants, I have been disappointed only once. And rarely have I actually been charged when there was no listed fruit that I could have ordered in the first place. I always leave an extra-large gratuity to show my appreciation. I imagine that more restaurants will offer fresh fruit desserts and begin to charge when more people begin to do as I do.

As I discuss more fully in the next chapter, your very best strategy to control calories when eating in restaurants, as well as at home, is to keep yourself out of the way of temptation. Keep whatever is not in your plan off the table, or, when dining with friends who want such foods, place these foods out of your reach. Make a public declaration that you will not be eating such and such at that meal. It will help you stick to your guns.

Why Whole Grains?

Many nutrients are lost in the milling of grains. Only a few (iron, thiamin, riboflavin, niacin) are replaced in the enrichment formulas used by food processors in making bread. Even these added nutrients may not be replaced in the flour used for desserts and pastries. Table 2 shows you how much nutritional value is missing from enriched refined wheat flour as compared with 100 percent whole wheat. As you can see in the case of most nutrients, one-half to three-quarters, or even more, of the nutrient content is lost. In addition to the loss of vitamins and minerals, you lose the fiber that contributes to healthy digestive processes and to some wasting of fat calories in the rest of your meal.

You won't be undernourished if you eat processed grains provided you also eat a wide variety of other foods. Beef and pork, for example, contain many of the same nutrients as whole grains. They cost a great deal more, however, and contain much more fat. But, if you eat white bread, you are getting a lot less nutrition per calorie and per dollar spent. Why waste money and calories this way?

TABLE 2

Nutrients in Enriched All-Purpose Flour Compared with Whole Wheat

(*per 150 Calories*)

NUTRIENT	WHOLE WHEAT	ALL PURPOSE	PERCENTAGE OF NUTRITIVE VALUE LOST IN MILLING
Calcium	18.47 mg	6.59 mg	−64%
Iron	1.49 mg	1.20 mg	−19%
Phosphorus	167.57 mg	35.85 mg	−79%
Potassium	166.67 mg	39.15 mg	−77%
Magnesium	67.66 mg	12.32 mg	−82%
Chromium	2.25 mg	1.24 mg	−45%
Manganese	2207.21 mg	247.25 mg	−89%
Cobalt	33.78 mg	14.84 mg	−56%
Copper	183.78 mg	61.81 mg	−66%
Zinc	1.40 mg	0.37 mg	−74%
Molybdenum	35.59 mg	13.19 mg	−63%

Source: Food and Nutrition News, Vol. 51, No. 5, 1980.

If you decide to switch to whole grain bread, be sure to read the label. Many breads that say *"Contains* 100 percent whole wheat flour" or products *"made with* 100 percent whole wheat flour" or made with some certain number of "natural grains," are really made primarily with all-purpose flour, a small amount of whole grain, and possibly a little coloring to make them look like whole wheat. If a bread is truly 100 percent whole wheat, it must say pure and simple "100 percent whole wheat."

Do You Need Vitamin Supplements?

You need not waste your money on unnecessary vitamin-mineral supplementation when you follow the dietary principles contained in the Double Your Fat Loss Diet. Your body will not absorb the water soluble vitamins if you don't need them; you simply flush them down the toilet. And the fat soluble vitamins can be stored in your body organs up to a point where they can cause serious illness, even death.

Nutrient supplementation is needed only by those persons who follow unsound, low calorie diets, for an extended period of time, or who have special physical problems that are rightly cared for by their physicians. Other exceptions include heavy smokers, who may need additional vitamin C, individuals who use a great deal of alcohol and coffee, who may need more B vitamins, and women on oral contraceptives, who may need more of both.

I suggest vitamin and mineral supplementation only to people whose food preferences or allergies make it impossible to consume a wide variety of foods, or to those few individuals who must reduce their caloric intake below the level I recommend in this book in order to achieve a satisfactory weight loss. In no case do I believe you should take more than a standard, balanced-formula, multiple vitamin-mineral supplement (about 100 percent of the Recommended Dietary Allowances) without your physician's supervision. Possible toxic effects result from high doses, and if you load your body with unnecessary vitamins and minerals, you may lower its naturally given ability to utilize nutrients efficiently. You may come to require large doses and suffer rebound deficiencies when you stop taking them.

There is no substitute for sound nutrition. That's what you get when you reduce your fat calorie consumption and increase fruits, vegetables, and whole grains along with the amounts of calcium and protein foods that I recommend.

Diet Drinks Can Destroy Your Diet

Do you have a sweet tooth? Are you substituting diet drinks for sugar-sweetened soft drinks? Do you still yearn for the real thing and find yourself eating other highly sweetened foods such as candy and desserts, if not frequently, then in very large quantities once you let go? If so, you are not doing yourself a favor with diet drinks (or by using large amounts of artificial sweeteners in other foods, as many diet cookbooks urge you to do). You are only keeping alive a need for sweeteners which, for you, may end up being associated with both a high sugar and a high fat consumption.

I have never yet worked with an overweight person for whom diet drinks served as an aid to weight control. Of course, I see a special group of people who have trouble controlling their weight. Some are drinking two to six or even more diet drinks a day and they are still fat. Combined with their inactivity, it's the other sugar-sweetened foods such as chocolate (which often has 60 percent of its caloric content in fat) as well as pies, cakes, and cookies (often 40 to 50 percent fat calories) in which they indulge at other times that are responsible. These individuals find that diet drinks don't always satisfy their desire for sweets. On certain occasions the diet drink itself seems to set off an urge for sweetness that only sugar foods can satisfy.

The destructive role that diet drinks can play is beautifully illustrated by one of my overweight diabetic patients. Her physician encouraged the use of diet drinks in an effort to control her addiction to sweets. I was not going to insist otherwise until I saw some eating records and was sure of my ground. Sure enough, she drank approximately thirty-six ounces of diet cola a day for three, four, even five or six days. But then came a binge, usually on chocolate or chocolate fudge, but chocolate cake also filled the bill. Until she eliminated all diet drinks and intensely artificially sweetened foods (using the technique I describe in chapter eleven), she could neither control her diabetic condition nor her yen for sweets.

My advice to you is to do the same as this diabetic patient.

If you resist that advice but your behavior is at all similar to the patient I've just described, then I suggest you do the following experiment which will settle the issue either in my favor or in yours.

Ask yourself whether you really crave that diet cola at certain times of the day. Could you give it up without a second thought? Try water or tea the next time you would ordinarily have a diet drink and if you still crave the sweetness and flavor of that diet cola, then face it. You've been hooked. I win.

Get rid of those diet drinks and then you, too, will be a winner in your battle with your sweet tooth. You are, in fact, much better off drinking fruit juices in spite of their few calories. Or have a piece of fruit and a glass of water. Instead of chemicals and caffeine, you'll be putting the nutrients that nature intended you to have in your body. By using fruit and fruit juices in place of diet drinks, you can reduce your drive for sugar-sweetened foods. And by keeping your hunger within bounds, fruit snacks will reduce any tendency to overeat at meals.

Using Alcohol

Because alcohol provides only empty calories and is immediately burned and used for energy by the body, it allows any surplus calories from other foods to be converted to fat. If you use more than a modest amount of alcohol, you may find it very hard to lose weight. Not only are you taking in too many empty calories, but after a couple of drinks, you may find yourself eating a lot more of everything else without realizing it or caring. That is, until the next day.

If you tend to use alcohol at the end of the work day, part of the problem is licked if that is the time you plan your activity. Then, to quench your thirst you can have a variety of substitute drinks available. Head straight for the water, herb tea, or some diluted fruit juice.

Because alcohol has no nutritional value except for its calories, you cannot substitute it for nourishing food in a reducing regimen. It must be consumed in addition to the healthful diet I have recommended. In most cases, the maximum amount of alcohol that seems possible to include in a diet, without deleterious effects, is one drink per day for a woman, two for a man. You can add that amount and hardly slow your weight loss at all. However, you can always do what one of my patients did—she added an extra fifteen minutes of walking each day to compensate for the glass of wine she planned to enjoy at dinner. She still lost about two pounds a week.

If you have been drinking more than two servings of alcoholic beverages a day, I think you are going to be pleasantly surprised when you drop it from your diet completely or cut down to one or two servings. You may find, as have many of my patients, that you sleep a lot better, feel much better when you get up in the morning, and perform better in any strenuous or skilled physical activity.

After you reach desirable weight, alcohol in moderation will not make an active person fat. In fact, on the average, runners tend to drink considerably more beer than non-runners and they certainly do not get fat. For many people nothing quite matches a cold beer after a long run or tennis match at the end of the day. You, too, can look forward to it without fear of gaining weight again if you have become an active person.

How Long Do You Diet?

Successful weight losers have a plan. Either they set a weight loss goal and stick to their diet until they reach it, or they decide on a period of time during which they adhere to their plan *regardless of how much weight they lose*. Then they enter a period of weight maintenance, confident that they will not regain their weight because of their new active lifestyle. I generally prefer this second approach.

If you have more than twenty-five or thirty pounds to lose, I suggest you decide on a set period of time for caloric restriction. It should be between a minimum of three weeks and a maximum of three months. Although the diet I recommend is nutritionally sound and can be used for an extended period of time, very few people can stick to a reduced caloric intake for more than three months.

Even if you have fifty pounds to lose, or seventy as I did, you will find it physically and psychologically less demanding, and less taxing on your friends and family, to build in some times out from dieting. You can be flexible. Either before you begin, at the three-week point, or at any point thereafter, decide when you will take that time out. This will give you an opportunity to experiment with increasing your caloric intake and determine to what extent your new activity level controls your weight. Weigh yourself every day. Expect as much as a two- or three-pound initial gain which tends to occur when a person goes off any diet. It's the added water involved in and produced by the metabolism of more food. Just one or two big meals can do it. You should hold fairly steady after that initial gain. However, do not allow yourself to put on more than two or three pounds without taking remedial action. If you begin to creep up, you have probably added too much fat and sugar to your diet.

I never dieted more than four weeks at a time during the period when I lost my own surplus weight. It took about a year and a half. Several times I took a respite from my diet and enjoyed eating and drinking just as much as I wanted, *after my daily tennis match.* It's true that I have a few star patients who have dieted continuously twelve to eighteen months until they have lost as much as 125 pounds. They are the exceptions. Many others set that high goal, in spite of my advice. At around the three-month mark they find themselves enjoying their new activities but getting tired of constantly watching their food intake.

If you have more weight to lose than can comfortably be taken off in a three-month period, plan for a time out right from the start. You will find it's good for your morale. After a few weeks vacation, you will be eager to get back on your diet and your enthusiasm will return as you watch your weight loss accelerate once again.

Insuring Your Success

Many people decide that it's time to diet and begin without making a single preparation to insure its success. Soon, just as with their vows to get active, all the antagonistic environmental and interpersonal forces, as well as their own established habits, overwhelm their good intentions and they fail once again.

You can help yourself succeed by preparing your family, your friends, and the environment around you, including your pantry, your refrigerator, and your office desk to become your allies instead of your enemies. Some of the more successful strategies are discussed in greater detail in the next chapter, but for now, in order to get started, you should make the following preparations. Check them off as you complete them.

DIETER'S CHECKLIST
Seven Steps to Success

1. Inform your family of your plans. Explain the program, the nature of your diet, and how you will fit your plans into the family's eating pattern. ( ) ——————————

2. Make up a shopping list and purchase the food you plan to eat this week. Plenty of fruits, vegetables, and the particular cuts of meat, fish, and fowl. See that you have a large selection of herbs for the experiment with seasonings. ( ) ——————————

3. Pick out a special selection of fruits and vegetables that you will use as substitutes for high calorie snacks and desserts. If you are a problem eater, read chapter eleven and plan your behavior change strategies. ( ) ——————————

4. Inform your friends and office colleagues of your plan. See if someone will join you in your effort (both diet and activity). Ask your friends to avoid tempting you to change your diet until you are ready to change. ( ) ——————————

5. Set up a plan for the meals you must eat away from home. Be prepared to bring lunch or get an agreement from at least one friend to go with you to restaurants where you can obtain low calorie meals. Always have a fruit that you can carry with you to work to substitute for high calorie snacks. ( ) ——————————

6. Do not accept dinner invitations at someone else's home without explaining that you are following this diet. Tell them you will be glad to bring your own meal just to enjoy their company, if their menu is not consistent with your plan. Be firm: deviate only during a planned time out.   ( ) _____

7. Do not begin to diet unless you have already begun to implement your program of physical activity. Are you setting aside the time *every day*?   ( ) _____

After Your Diet: Weight Maintenance

Once they have reached goal weight, most active weight losers never need to diet again. But a small minority of my seriously overweight readers will have developed eating habits for which no reasonable amount of activity can counterbalance. If you happen to be one of these individuals, remember this motto, "You can't get fat if you eat no fat."

Of course, fat is an essential nutrient—you must have a small amount of fat in your diet to supply essential fatty acids and transport the fat soluble vitamins, A, D, E, and K. I phrase my motto in the extreme, however, to keep you conscious of the fact that the major culprit in obesity, when caloric intake is at fault and not a sedentary lifestyle, is an overconsumption of fat. It's not the oft-blamed starchy foods such as bread, beans, and pasta, but what goes on them that hurts. Even in candy and desserts, it's that 40 to 60 percent fat calories, combined with the sugar and corn syrup, that do the damage. So, unless you are addicted to sugar-laden soft drinks or alcohol and consume several drinks per day, it's usually your fat consumption that must be controlled.

If you find yourself slowly regaining weight after you've reached your goal and established the level of activity that will keep most formerly sedentary individuals slim and fit for life, then take another look at your fat consumption. Odds are you will have been deviating from the dietary principles that I have outlined in this chapter. If you always trim and skim visible fats, avoid fried foods and snacks, and never use more than the minimum amounts of additional fat that I suggest for cooking and flavor in my Seven-Day Plan, I think you will find that you can eat quite freely in every other way. By keeping fat intake low, you eliminate the major source of surplus calories in your diet.

RECIPES

Main Dishes

This selection of main dish recipes illustrates how well you can eat and still control your weight. As you prepare these recipes you will learn a style of cooking suitable for all occasions. You don't have to cook one way for yourself, another for your family, and yet another for company.

Alternate and substitute these main dish recipes with the ones given in the Seven-Day Plan.

When the full recipes are divided into the suggested serving sizes, each serving of the fish and fowl dishes will contain approximately 175 to 200 calories. The meat dishes will contain approximately 250 to 350 calories, with the ones at the higher end of this range having cheese as well as meat as an ingredient.

Tender Marinated Round Steak

1½ lbs. round steak, ¾ to 1 inch thick
½ cup soy sauce
¼ cup water (or dry red table wine)
1 clove garlic, minced
2 tablespoons bell pepper flakes
2 tablespoons dehydrated minced onion
½ teaspoon ground ginger

Marinate meat and other ingredients in refrigerator for three hours or overnight. Turn at least once. Broil over charcoal or under broiler, basting before turning.

This is an all-purpose marinade and can be used to advantage with pork chops and lamb. The tougher the cut of meat, the longer it should be marinated.

Marinades do not need extra sugar. You can experiment with adding other ingredients such as one teaspoon worcestershire sauce, one teaspoon chopped chives, or two tablespoons chopped scallions. Sherry (⅛ cup) can also be used in place of the water or wine to impart a sweeter flavor. Serves four.

Baked Pork Chops

4 loin chops, well-trimmed,
approximately 1 inch thick
whole wheat flour for dredging
garlic powder and salt to taste
2 teaspoons olive oil

½ teaspoon dried basil
½ cup sherry (Madeira or Marsala) wine, (apricot or plum juice can be substituted for wine)

Preheat oven to 250°. Combine flour, garlic powder, and salt in plastic baggie. Add chops and shake until they are thoroughly coated. Brown in heavy skillet with oil. Arrange chops in shallow baking dish. Sprinkle with basil and cover with aluminum foil. Bake until chops are tender (about 1½ hours). Remove cover. Skim off all fat. Add wine or fruit juice and continue baking, uncovered, until liquid bubbles. Baste occasionally. Serves four.

Beef-Eggplant Casserole

2 large eggplants, sliced ½ inch thick (peeling optional)
1 large onion, chopped
1 large green pepper, chopped
2 teaspoons oil
1 pound lean ground round beef
1 tablespoon whole wheat flour

1 teaspoon salt
½ teaspoon oregano
½ teaspoon basil
2½ cups tomato sauce
garlic powder and freshground pepper to taste
1½ cups parmesan cheese

Steam eggplant in ½ cup salted water until barely tender. Brown onion and green pepper in oil. Remove from pan and brown meat. Remove meat from pan with a slotted spoon and pour off any remaining fat. Return beef, onions, and peppers to pan and add flour, spices, and tomato sauce. Cook until it starts to thicken. In a large casserole, layer one-half the eggplant, one-half the sauce, and one-half the cheese. Repeat with the remainder and bake at 325° for 35–45 minutes. Serves six.

The next dish has the flavor of meat and legumes that have been cooked with ham hocks or salt pork, but it has only a fraction of the fat. If you have ever doubted that you can have that special flavor without fat, be sure to try this dish. It can also be made with lamb shanks, or beef brisket in place of veal.

Veal with Lentils

Rinse 1½ cup lentils and soak in water overnight. Next day add to lentils and the liquid: 1 onion stuck with 2 cloves, 1 bayleaf, and 1 teaspoon salt. Bring to boil, then turn down and simmer until just tender. Let lentils cool in their own liquid. (Lentils will take 35–45 minutes to cook.)

2 pounds boned veal roast, trimmed	2 cloves garlic, minced
½ cup whole wheat flour	½ teaspoon salt
2 teaspoons oil	fresh ground pepper to taste
dry mustard	1 cup meat broth (or ½ cup broth,
ginger	and ½ cup dry white or table
oregano	wine)
tarragon	soy sauce

Cut veal roast into six pieces while lentils are simmering. Toss meat in bag containing flour until well coated. Brown in oil, sprinkling each side of meat with small amounts of dry mustard, ginger, oregano, and tarragon. Add garlic, salt, pepper, and broth (or wine mixture). Sprinkle with a few drops of soy sauce and simmer, covered, until tender. Drain lentils and reserve liquid. Remove cloves and chop onions. Place lentils and chopped onions in casserole, top with meat, and add all pan juices plus lentil liquid until combined liquid covers the tops of the lentils. Bake uncovered at 375° for forty minutes. Serves six.

Quick Corn Beef and Cabbage

On your way home, pick up one-half to one pound of thinly sliced lean corn beef from the delicatessen.

Trim and wedge cabbage. Steam in small amount of water in covered saucepan for about fifteen minutes or until just fork-tender. Cabbage is best when it is rather crisp and not overcooked. Drain and season with salt and pepper and small amount of butter if desired. To serve, lay strips of precooked corn beef over hot cabbage wedges. Serves four.

Chili Con Carne

1 tablespoon butter or oil	½ teaspoon cayenne
1 large white onion, chopped	1 teaspoon cumin
3 cloves garlic, finely minced	1 medium bayleaf
1 pound lean ground round steak	2 tablespoons Mexican-style chili
1 large can peeled tomatoes	powder
(approximately 28 ounces)	¼ teaspoon basil
1 fifteen-ounce can tomato sauce	1 teaspoon salt
1 green pepper, chopped	1 twelve-ounce can red kidney
½ teaspoon celery seed	beans

Heat butter in skillet. Add onion, garlic, and green pepper, and sauté until they begin to brown. Add meat and brown.

Transfer mixture to large saucepan with slotted spoon, leaving any fat behind. Add all remaining ingredients except beans. Bring to a boil, reduce heat, and simmer uncovered until sauce approaches desired thickness (from forty-five minutes to an hour). Add kidney beans, including liquid just before serving. Mash approximately one-half the beans into the mixture to impart flavor and further thicken the sauce. Delicious with grated cheddar, swiss, gruyère, or parmesan cheese. Serves six.

Spicy Meat Loaf

1 pound lean ground round steak	1 cup tomato sauce
2 eggs beaten	1 tablespoon prepared horserad-
2 medium white onions, chopped	ish
1 medium green pepper, chopped	1 teaspoon dry mustard
2 stalks celery, minced	¼ teaspoon garlic powder
2 medium carrots, grated	½ teaspoon salt
1 tablespoon chopped fresh pars-	½ teaspoon freshly ground pep-
ley (1 teaspoon dry)	per

Preheat oven to 350°. Mix all ingredients and place in lightly greased baking pan. Bake for one hour and drain any fat before serving. Serves four.

Quick Italian Meatloaf

1 pound lean ground round steak
¼ cup dried herb flavored bread-
    crumbs
2 teaspoons soy sauce
¼ teaspoon oregano
1 teaspoon worcestershire
1 egg
1 fifteen-ounce can tomato sauce
freshly ground pepper

Combine all ingredients except tomato sauce. Place in baking dish and bake at 350° about thirty minutes. Pour off fat and cover loaf with tomato sauce. Bake for another thirty minutes. Serves four.

Lemon Baked Chicken

1 three-pound fryer, cut up
3 tablespoons fresh lemon juice
garlic powder, fresh ground pep-
    per, salt to taste
chopped parsley

Preheat oven to 350°. Arrange chicken in shallow casserole or baking dish. Pour lemon juice over the chicken, spreading it if necessary with your fingertips to get an even coating. Sprinkle with garlic powder, salt, and pepper. Cover and bake about forty-five minutes. Uncover and brown for an additional ten minutes. To serve, remove skin, and sprinkle with parsley. Serves four.

Baked Herb Chicken

1 three-pound fryer, cut up
4 small onions, cooked (boiled) or
    2 medium-sized onions finely
    chopped, uncooked
1 large carrot, chopped
2 tablespoons fresh parsley,
    chopped (or 2 teaspoons dried)
½ teaspoon thyme leaves
¼ teaspoon celery seed
½ teaspoom tarragon
½ cup fresh mushrooms sliced
1 cup dry white table wine
1 bayleaf
garlic powder, salt, and pepper
    to taste

Brown chicken in hot fat. Sprinkle with salt, pepper, and garlic powder and place in casserole dish. Drain excess fat from skillet and heat remaining ingredients for about two minutes, scraping up brown pieces. Pour over chicken. Cover and bake at 350° for seventy-five to ninety minutes or until fork-tender. Serves four.

Barbecued Chicken

3 pounds chicken breasts and thighs, washed and skinned
2 tablespoons vinegar
2 tablespoons worcestershire sauce
1 teaspoon chili powder
½ teaspoon cayenne
3 tablespoons ketchup
1 tablespoon lemon juice
4 tablespoons water
1 teaspoon dry mustard
1 teaspoon paprika
2 tablespoons dry sherry (optional)

Place chicken on heavy foil, allowing plenty to fold over, and set to the side. Combine remaining ingredients and cook over low heat until blended. Pour sauce over chicken, coating each piece well. Fold up foil so that chicken and sauce are sealed. Place on cookie sheet and bake at 450° for fifteen minutes. Reduce heat to 350° and bake one hour longer. Serve with sauce poured over chicken. Leftovers are delicious cold. Serves eight.

Fish Fillets in White Wine

1 pound fillets (flounder, turbot, cod, pollack, or other)
2 tomatoes, sliced
½ cup dry white table wine
½ teaspoon basil
½ teaspoon parsley
salt and fresh ground pepper to taste
½ cup freshly grated cheddar cheese

Lightly salt and pepper fillets on both sides and place in baking dish. Arrange tomatoes on top. Add wine and sprinkle with herbs. Bake at 350° for twenty minutes. Sprinkle with cheese and bake about five minutes longer until fish flakes with fork. Serves four.

Crisp Baked Rainbow Trout (or fish fillets)

4 small trout (up to ¾ pounds each) or 1-pound fish fillets
¼ cup seasoned French or Italian salad dressing
1 cup fine dry bread crumbs (or ½ cup whole wheat flour for dredging)

Preheat oven to 500°. Dip fish into salad dressing and then into bread crumbs (or shake in baggie with whole wheat flour until well coated). Arrange fish on lightly oiled foil-lined baking pan. Bake about twelve minutes or until fish flakes with fork. Serves four.

Fish Skillet

1 pound fish fillets or steaks
1 tablespoon vegetable oil or butter
1 medium onion, chopped
1 small green pepper, chopped
2 tablespoons fresh parsley, chopped (2 teaspoons dried)

2 medium tomatoes, sliced
1 seven-ounce can minced clams
½ teaspoon basil or oregano
fresh ground pepper to taste

Heat fat in skillet and add all vegetables except tomatoes. Cook covered until onion is soft and transparent, about five minutes on medium heat. Add tomatoes and seasonings. Cook until soft. Add fish and clams. Cover and simmer gently until fish flakes easily with fork (approximately fifteen minutes). If more liquid is needed during cooking, water, tomato juice, V-8 juice, or dry white table wine can be added. Serves four.

The following illustrates how delicious high calorie dishes can be adapted to low fat cooking. The original recipe calls for 1½ cups mayonnaise, which contain approximately 2400 calories. This adaptation, which replaces the mayonnaise with cream of shrimp soup, saves 2000 calories, or 250 calories per serving.

Seafood Casserole

1 package (6 ozs. frozen crab meat)
2 cups cooked shrimp (approximately 8 ounces frozen)
2 cups diced celery
1 medium onion, chopped
4 hard-boiled eggs, diced

1 cup fresh mushrooms, sliced
1 can sliced water chestnuts
salt to taste
2 cans cream of shrimp soup
½ cup toasted bread crumbs
½ cup slivered almonds

Thaw and drain crab meat and shrimp. Mix all ingredients except bread crumbs and almonds in a large baking dish. When thoroughly blended, top with bread crumbs and almonds. Bake at 350° for about forty-five minutes. This casserole is delicious over rice. Serves eight.

Broiled Salmon Steaks with Herbs

4 salmon steaks, 1 to 1½ inches thick
1 tablespoon oil
2 tablespoons dry white wine
juice of one-half lemon
thyme, marjoram, sage, salt and fresh ground pepper to taste

Pour oil and wine, and squeeze lemon juice onto a foil-lined broiling pan. Rub fish steaks in the mixture and coat both sides evenly. Sprinkle both sides of the fish lightly with herbs (leaves or powders). Salt and pepper to taste. Broil two inches to three inches from flame for 5 to 7½ minutes on each side. Serves four.

Vegetables

These sixteen recipes for cooked vegetables have been selected to illustrate low fat but still flavorful ways of cooking. *No recipe contains more than 25 calories of added fat per serving.* Begin to adapt all of your own recipes for cooked vegetables to contain no more than one tablespoon of fat for a four-serving recipe.

If a vegetable can be eaten raw, it generally retains more of its nutritional value. Much of the water-soluble vitamin content of vegetables (B-complex vitamins and vitamin C) and possibly some minerals will be lost to the cooking water or actually destroyed in cooking. Therefore, save your vegetable stock for soups and for cooking rice or boiling potatoes. And plan to eat some vegetables raw every day in a salad or as a snack. In addition to carrot sticks and celery, cauliflower, broccoli, cucumbers, radishes, yellow crookneck squash, tomatoes, and zucchini make for good low calorie nibbling. I especially recommend small, fresh, tender yellow squash. They are sweet and very filling.

Baked Asparagus with Cheese

24 asparagus spears, cooked
lemon juice
4 ounces thinly sliced gruyère or swiss cheese
4 tablespoons freshly grated parmesan cheese

Preheat oven to 400°. Arrange a layer of asparagus in a lightly greased baking dish. Sprinkle with lemon juice. Partially cover the asparagus with slices of cheese and lightly sprinkle with parmesan. Repeat layers, ending with cheese. Bake until cheese is melted and bubbling—about ten minutes. Serves four.

Green Beans with Water Chestnuts

Sauté one-half cup drained and coarsely chopped water chestnuts in one tablespoon butter for three minutes. Pour over two cups hot drained beans. Season to taste with salt, pepper, and a pinch of herbs (basil, chervil, or oregano). Serves four.

Minted Green Beans

4 tablespoons fresh mint leaves, chopped (2 teaspoons dried)
1 tablespoon butter
¼ teaspoon pepper
2 cups cooked green beans, drained

Combine beans with other ingredients and heat thoroughly. Serves four.

Lima Beans with Rosemary

Season two cups hot, drained lima beans with one tablespoon butter and one-quarter teaspoon dried rosemary. Salt and pepper to taste. Serves four.

Broccoli with Black Olives

1 bunch fresh broccoli (1½ pounds)
1 tablespoon olive oil
1 clove garlic, minced
¼ cup chopped, pitted, black olives
4 tablespoons freshly grated parmesan cheese
salt and pepper to taste

Cook broccoli in small amount of salted water for ten minutes. Drain. Sauté garlic in oil until lightly brown. Add broccoli, season with salt and pepper and cook over low heat about ten minutes, but do not overcook. Broccoli is best crisp. Add olives and heat thoroughly (two minutes). Serve immediately and sprinkle with cheese. Serves four.

Brussels Sprouts with Caraway Seeds

1 pound brussels sprouts (about
2½ cups)
water or chicken broth

1 tablespoon butter
salt and pepper to taste
1 teaspoon caraway seeds

Wash brussels sprouts and trim wilted leaves. Make a gash in the bottom of each to speed cooking. Place in one-half cup salted, boiling water or chicken broth, cover, reduce heat, and permit to steam until just fork-tender. Do not overcook. Pour off liquid and save as stock. Add butter, caraway seeds, and salt and pepper to taste. Serves four.

Cabbage and Celery Casserole

½ cup celery, chopped
2 tablespoons butter
3½ cups chopped cabbage
½ teaspoon salt
⅛ teaspoon freshly ground
pepper

1 cup white sauce
1 tablespoon chopped pimiento
¼ cup dry herb flavored bread
crumbs

Using large saucepan, cook celery in two teaspoons butter for ten minutes, stirring occasionally. Add cabbage, cover, and steam about ten minutes. Pour into baking dish, add salt, pepper, white sauce, and pimento. Sprinkle bread crumbs over top and bake at 350° for twenty minutes. Serves eight.

Cooked Carrots

Allow one pound carrots or approximately two cups for four servings. Wash, but do not scrape or peel. Cook covered in a small amount of salted, boiling water until fork-tender. I like my carrots either whole or in rather large pieces when their length exceeds the diameter of my pot. Season with salt and pepper and one tablespoon butter for four servings.

Carrots with Cheese Sauce

2 tablespoons melted butter
1 tablespoon low fat milk
3 tablespoons whole wheat flour
1½ cups milk
½ teaspoon salt
⅛ teaspoon freshly ground black
   pepper

dash cayenne
¾ cup grated cheese
3½ cups cooked carrots
pinch of rosemary

Blend butter and one tablespoon milk with flour. Add the rest of the milk slowly and cook until thickened, stirring constantly. Add seasonings and one-half cup of the cheese. Place carrots in baking dish. Cover with sauce and top with remaining cheese. Bake at 350° for fifteen minutes. Serves eight.

Cauliflower with Tasty Toppings

Steam cook a whole large head of cauliflower or bring to boil one-half cup water in large saucepan. Add cauliflower, cover, and reduce heat. Cook until fork-tender but be careful not to overcook (twenty-five to thirty minutes).

Place cauliflower in large serving bowl and top with one-quarter cup dried-herb-flavored bread crumbs that have been mixed with two tablespoons melted butter. Sprinkle with one diced hard-boiled egg and one tablespoon fresh parsley, chopped. Serves six to eight.

Greens in White, Egg, or Cheese Sauce

Mix four cups cooked greens (for example, collards, dandelions, kale, mustard, spinach, or turnip) with one recipe white, egg, or cheese sauce. Heat thoroughly in saucepan on top of stove or in casserole in oven for twenty minutes at 350°. Serves eight.

Seasoned Mushrooms on Toast

In large heavy skillet, simmer one pound whole mushrooms in two tablespoons butter, two tablespoons soy sauce, and one teaspoon worcestershire until mushrooms are hot and slightly brown. Do not overcook. Salt and pepper to taste. Serve on toast, covering with remaining sauce from pan. The mushrooms can be flamed in one ounce of brandy before serving. Serves four.

Marinated Mushrooms

Marinate one-half pound of whole mushrooms in one-quarter cup Italian dressing. Use double plastic baggies, well tied, since baggies frequently develop a leak. Mix the mushrooms around in the marinade every few hours.

This makes a tasty low-calorie hors d'oeuvre served raw. It can be broiled in the oven, or grilled over charcoal. It's an excellent accompaniment to steak.

Sautéed Tomatoes

Choose two good-sized (three-inch diameter) firm tomatoes. Slice, dip into beaten egg, and then into dry, seasoned breadcrumbs. Sprinkle with salt and pepper and an additional pinch of basil or oregano. Brown on both sides in one tablespoon melted butter or olive oil in heavy skillet. Serves four.

Greens Casserole

1 pound chopped greens (spinach, kale, collards, or broccoli)
3 eggs
6 tablespoons whole wheat flour
½ teaspoon each salt and oregano
ground pepper to taste
3 tablespoons wheat germ

Beat eggs and flour together until smooth. Add everything but the wheat germ. Mix well and pour into baking dish about 8 x 12 inches in size. Sprinkle wheat germ over the top and bake uncovered at 350° for approximately forty-five minutes.

Fresh or frozen greens may be used. If fresh are used, cook them in a small amount of water until wilted before combining in the casserole.

For variety, add two cups grated cheddar cheese to mixture before pouring into baking pan.

Two- or Three-Squash Casserole

Pick up a variety of summer squash—yellow, white button, zucchini—whatever is available. Figure one medium yellow squash or zucchini per person; a medium-sized (five-inch) white button squash will do for two. The following recipe serves six.

2 each yellow squash and zucchini, about five to six inches
long
1 5-inch white button (or two small
three-inch pattypans)
1 large (twenty-nine-ounce) can
tomato sauce

1 cup freshly grated parmesan
cheese
garlic and onion powder
freshly ground pepper

Cut the squash into one-half inch slices and place in saucepan with one-half cup boiling water. Sprinkle lightly with garlic and onion powder and freshly ground pepper. Cover tightly and cook until squash is just barely tender. It should be hot, but still crunchy. It is better to undercook than to overcook. Drain well.

Preheat oven to 350°. Place half the squash in deep pie pan or casserole. Cover with half the tomato sauce and half the grated cheese. Repeat the layers. Bake until the cheese is bubbly and beginning to brown.

Low Calorie White, Egg, and Cheese Sauces for Vegetables

Almost any vegetable alone, or in your favorite combinations can be cooked with my low calorie, but rich-tasting, white sauce, which adds only 60 calories per serving. By using one of these sauces, you increase the value of the incomplete proteins that are found in vegetables. You also add some calcium to your meal.

Use four cups cooked vegetables to serve eight, with one recipe of the sauces. Just add the sauce to cooked, drained vegetables and heat thoroughly on top of the stove, or bake the mixture in a casserole for twenty minutes at 350°.

Try these sauces with broccoli, brussels sprouts, carrots, cauliflower, celery, green beans, kale, lima beans, mushrooms, onions, parsnips, peas, spinach, and other greens.

Basic White Sauce

2 tablespoons butter	2 cups low fat milk
1 tablespoon low fat milk	½ teaspoon salt
3 tablespoons whole wheat flour	⅛ teaspoon pepper

Melt butter. Add one tablespoon low fat milk and stir in flour. When blended, add the two cups of milk gradually, and cook slowly until thickened. Add salt and pepper. Makes two cups of sauce or enough to serve eight when combined with vegetables.

Cheese Sauce

Stir one-half cup grated cheese into the sauce.

Egg Sauce

Add chopped whites and mashed yolks of two hard-cooked eggs and one teaspoon minced parsley to sauce.

Festive Fruit Salads

Tasty and attractive fruit salads are easy to prepare. You will have discovered by using my examples in the Seven-Day Plan that adding just a small amount of protein and fat from nuts, seeds, or a bit of cheese can make fruit salads very satisfying. They also become much more nutritious with these additions.

For festive fruit salads, start with any fruit which has a shell you can use for serving such as a pineapple or a melon. Slice in half. (Cut a pineapple lengthwise without removing the leaf spikes to make an attractive serving vessel.) Remove the meat from the shell and cut into bite-size pieces. Reserve shell.

Choosing whatever is in season, cut up a selection of your favorite fresh fruits, such as pears, peaches, plums, apples, and berries. Combine with the melon or pineapple in a large mixing bowl. Add a small amount of fresh lemon or orange juice to preserve color and add tartness.

As for quantity, I find that a whole pineapple, cantaloupe, or small honeydew melon, combined with two peaches, two pears, and one and a half to two cups each of blueberries and sliced strawberries will easily serve four. To this quantity I add a total of eight tablespoons of any combination raisins, cut-up dates, or figs, and four tablespoons of any combination shredded coconut, nuts, or seeds.

To serve, return to the shells, or spoon over a large lettuce leaf on individual platters. Top each serving with a scoop (four tablespoons) cottage cheese, or one-half cup low fat yogurt. Total calories will usually equal about 300 per generous serving.

Experiment with making festive fruit salads and then, when you are ready to take your first time out from dieting, invite some friends to join you on a Sunday walk. When you all return home, pop open a bottle of really dry champagne (brut or natural), pour one glass over the fruit as you mix it, and enjoy the remaining champagne with your salad.

I particularly like champagne with melon, peaches, pineapple, and strawberries. For a large fruit salad, I start with a watermelon and use both honeydew and cantaloupe, as well as other fruit. Pile it all back into the watermelon shell. It makes for a colorful sight on an especially festive occasion. Use it for cocktail parties and buffets, with multicolored toothpicks dotting the top layer and a supply on the side. Use only ingredients that can be picked up with a toothpick when you prepare fruit this way, and serve nuts and cheese separately.

Hearty Soups

Any one of these three hearty soup recipes can serve as a complete nutritious meal. Each will contain between 150 and 200 calories per eight-ounce serving.

This barley soup recipe is like the one my mother used to make. She got it from her mother. It warmed me on cold winter nights when I was a child growning up in upstate New York.

Old Country Barley Soup

2 pounds trimmed soup meat or marrow bones
1 cup dried baby lima beans
¾ cup pearl barley
½ cup lentils

2 medium onions, diced
3 carrots, diced
3 stalks celery, diced
2 tablespoons salt
4 quarts water

Boil water, bones, or meat, and salt until a scum forms. Skim and add vegetables. Simmer 1½ hours in a covered pot. You can freeze half of this recipe and save it for another occasion.

Lentil Soup

We prepare many variations of lentil soup. This one is my wife's favorite.

1 cup lentils, rinsed and soaked overnight
2 large onions, chopped
1 carrot, chopped
2 teaspoons oil
½ teaspoon each thyme, marjoram, and basil
ground pepper and salt to taste

3 cups bouillon (use the water in which the lentils were soaked as part of this)
¼ cup fresh chopped parsley (2 tablespoons dried)
1 pound canned tomatoes
grated cheese of your choice (about 2 tablespoons per serving)

Sauté onions and carrots in the oil for three to five minutes. Add herbs and sauté a minute longer. Add the rest of the ingredients except the cheese and cook about forty-five minutes, covered, until lentils are tender. Put grated cheese at the bottom of each bowl, add soup, and serve. Serves six.

All sorts of beans and vegetables can be combined to make a delicious hearty soup. You can use your imagination and have a pleasant surprise with each recipe. Here is another that, in spite of similar ingredients, tastes quite different from the ones before.

Many Beans Soup

2 pounds lean soup meat
6 cups water
2 medium onions, diced
2 carrots, diced
3 stalks celery, diced
½ cup navy beans
½ cup lentils
⅓ cup soya grits

½ cup raw or canned garbanzos
1 teaspoon fresh dill weed (¼ teaspoon dried)
1 tablespoon salt
1 teaspoon mixed salad or Italian style blended herbs
1 teaspoon garlic powder

Boil water, meat, and salt, and skim scum. Add other ingredients and cook for approximately 1½ hours on low heat in a covered pot.

Miscellaneous

Meat Sauce for Pasta

1 pound lean ground round steak
1 large onion, chopped fine
1 stalk celery, chopped fine
1 green pepper, chopped fine
1 can (28 ounces) peeled tomatoes
1 small can (6 ounces) tomato paste

1 tablespoon worcestershire
1 teaspoon chili powder
½ teaspoon oregano
½ teaspoon basil
salt and pepper to taste

Brown first four ingredients and pour off any fat. Add remaining ingredients. Bring to a boil. Reduce heat and simmer uncovered for one to two hours or until sauce reaches desired thickness. Serve over hot cooked whole wheat pasta for a very healthy low calorie dish. One cup cooked spaghetti with three ounces of this sauce will contain approximately 325 calories.

All-Purpose Low Calorie Hot Barbecue Sauce

1 tablespoon vegetable oil
1 clove garlic, minced
½ cup ketchup
2 medium white onions, finely chopped

2 tablespoons vinegar
1 teaspoon dry mustard
½ teaspoon Tabasco

Mix in small saucepan and bring to a boil over medium heat. This sauce is good with all meats. The recipe makes one cup. Each tablespoon has approximately 10 calories.

GUIDE TO SEASONINGS

Allspice Meats, fish, gravies, relishes, tomato sauce

Anise Fruit

Basil Green beans, onions, peas, potatoes, summer squash, tomatoes, lamb, beef, shell fish, eggs, sauces

Bay Leaves Artichokes, beets, carrots, onions, white potatoes, tomatoes, meats, fish, soups and stews, sauces, and gravies

Caraway Seed Asparagus, beets, cabbage, carrots, cauliflower, cole slaw, onions, potatoes, sauerkraut, turnips, beef, pork, noodles, cheese dishes

Cardamon Melon, sweet potatoes

Cayenne Pepper Sauces, curries

Celery Seed Cabbage, carrots, cauliflower, corn, lima beans, potatoes, tomatoes, turnips, salad dressings, beef, fish dishes, sauces, soups, stews, cheese

Chervil Carrots, peas, salads, summer squash, tomatoes, salad dressings, poultry, fish, eggs

Chili Powder Corn, eggplant, onions, beef, pork, chili con carne, stews, shell fish, sauces, egg dishes

Chives Carrots, corn, sauces, salads, soups

Cinnamon Stewed fruits, apple or pineapple dishes, sweet potatoes, winter squash, toast

Cloves baked beans, sweet potatoes, winter squash, pork and ham roasts

Cumin Cabbage, rice, sauerkraut, chili con carne, ground beef dishes, cottage or cheddar cheese

Curry Powder Carrots, cauliflower, green beans, onions, tomatoes, pork and lamb, shell fish, fish, poultry, sauces for eggs and meats

Dill Seed Cabbage, carrots, cauliflower, peas, potatoes, spinach, tomato dishes, turnips, salads, lamb, cheese

Ginger Applesauce, melon, baked beans, carrots, onions, sweet potatoes, poultry, summer and winter squash, beef, veal, ham, lamb, teriyaki sauce

Mace Carrots, potatoes, spinach, summer squash, beef and veal, fruits, and sauces

Marjoram Asparagus, carrots, eggplant, greens, green beans, lima beans, peas, spinach, summer squash, lamb, pork, poultry, fish, stews, sauces

Mustard Asparagus, broccoli, Brussels sprouts, cabbage, cauliflower, green beans, onions, peas, potatoes, summer squash, meats, and poultry

Nutmeg Beets, Brussels sprouts, carrots, cabbage, cauliflower, greens, green beans, onions, spinach, sweet potatoes, winter squash, sauces

Oregano Baked beans, broccoli, cabbage, cauliflower, green beans, lima beans, onions, peas, potatoes, spinach, tomatoes, turnips, beef, pork, veal, poultry, fish, pizza, chili con carne, Italian sauces, stews

Paprika Salad dressings, shell fish, fish, gravies, eggs

Parsley Flakes All vegetables, soups, sauces, salads, stews, potatoes, eggs

Pepper Most vegetables, meats, salads

Poppy Seeds Salads, noodles

Rosemary Mushrooms, peas, potatoes, spinach, tomatoes, vegetable salads, beef, lamb, pork, veal, poultry, stews, cheese, and eggs

Sage Eggplant, onions, peas, tomato dishes and salads, pork, veal, poultry, ham, cheese

Saffron Rice

Savory Baked beans, beets, cabbage, carrots, cauliflower, lima beans, potatoes, rice, squash, egg dishes, roasts, and ground meat dishes

Sesame Seed Asparagus, green beans, potatoes, tomatoes, spinach

Tarragon Asparagus, beets, cabbage, carrots, cauliflower, mushrooms, tomatoes, salads, macaroni and vegetable combinations, beef, poultry, pork

Thyme Artichokes, beets, carrots, eggplant, green beans, mushrooms, peas, tomatoes, pork and veal, poultry, cheese and fish dishes, stuffings

Turmeric Mustards and curries, chicken

Cream-Style Low Calorie Salad Dressing

1 cup cottage cheese
½ cup buttermilk
salt, seasoned salt, and other flavors such as garlic and onion
powder or celery seed, to taste

1½ teaspoons lemon juice
1 tablespoon fresh chopped
parsley (1 teaspoon dried)

Mix cottage cheese in blender until smooth. Stir in buttermilk, lemon
juice, parsley, salt, and seasonings. Chill. Makes 1½ cups. Good on
baked potato, too. One tablespoon contains approximately 17 calories.

Corn Relish

1 can whole kernel corn, drained
¾ cup chopped celery
2 tablespoons chopped onion
2 tablespoons chopped green
pepper

1 tablespoon chopped pimiento
3 tablespoons wine vinegar
1 tablespoon prepared mustard
2 tablespoons pickle relish

Mix and chill. Each tablespoon contains approximately 12 calories.

Low Fat Brown Rice Pilaf

1 cup uncooked brown rice
1 cup chopped celery
2 medium white onions, chopped
½ cup fresh mushrooms, sliced

2 cups beef bouillon
1 tablespoon melted butter or oil
salt and pepper as desired

Preheat oven to 350°. Combine all ingredients in large casserole. Cover
and bake one hour.

This is an excellent base for a vegetable stir fry or a seafood casserole. You can also serve it in place of potatoes and bread.

The above method of cooking leads to rice that will stick together
slightly. To achieve a drier, nonsticky version, heat the uncooked grains
of rice in the fat over low heat until they begin to brown. Then proceed as above.

Leftover rice pilaf can be combined with leftover cooked vegetables such as kale, spinach, broccoli, carrots, peas, or beans and

made into a casserole. Mix your leftovers together with a blend of one egg, one-half to one cup milk (depending upon the quantity of leftovers), and add a dash of worcestershire. Top the mixture with coarsely grated sharp cheddar cheese and reheat at 350° for forty minutes.

One-half cup cooked rice pilaf will contain approximately 75 calories.

11

DOING AWAY WITH PROBLEM EATING

"When I have a box of cookies in the house I can resist for just so long. I finally eat one and then I can't stop until I finish them all."

"I'm a saint in public, but when I get home I go wild. I even sneak food after my family goes to bed."

If you have found yourself making statements like these, you may indeed have an eating drive for which reasonable activity can only partially compensate.

This chapter is devoted to helping you change poor eating habits and the situations that cause them. The strategies I describe have helped many people lose weight. Practice the ones that fit your eating problem while you are implementing your diet. Then, when you reach your goal weight and the level of activity that I recommend, you can continue to keep your eating under control with any changes in your environment or your behavior that you have already found to be useful.

Making Changes in Eating Behavior and the Eating Environment

Much of our behavior is strongly subject to environmental influences. Often we make unthinking, automatic responses and never pay attention to the control our environment exerts over us. We notice the control only when we make an effort to change. The following two simple events afford good illustrations of the forces at work in the more complex situations involving eating.

For example, the telephone rings. We answer it. We don't have to answer it, but most of the time we want to. Almost all of us have times, however, when we have things we need to do and prefer not to talk on the telephone. It's at times like these that we experience the power a ringing phone has over our behavior. It is extremely hard to resist answering. Once we answer it, we must either find a way to cut the conversation short or face not getting our other tasks done. The same type of situation occurs with television. We may be in the midst of some job we want to finish when we happen to wander through a room in which someone is watching an interesting program. We stop to watch for a moment only to be sucked into an hour or two of viewing.

Overeaters respond to the presence of certain foods like most of us respond to the telephone or a few minutes of TV viewing. If the food is present, or attracts our attention, we eat it. Once we start we might not be able to stop until we've eaten far more than we originally intended when we took that first taste.

We have three options when it comes to reducing the control the environment exerts over our behavior.

1. We can try to "guts it out." We can decide to force ourselves to ignore the cues in our environment that have some power over us and hope our *desire* to respond, as well as our actual response, will, in psychological terms, "extinguish."

2. We can change the saliency of the stimulus—disguise it, hide it, or otherwise reduce its ability to gain our attention and influence us.

3. We can completely rid the environment of the objects to which we have been reacting. This makes a response to those objects impossible.

Continuing the analogy with simple events, how can we apply these three approaches to the telephone situation? We can decide to ignore it and let it ring. Most likely, we will succeed a certain small portion of the time. We can remove the receiver from the hook so that it cannot ring. This reduces its saliency in our environment and we would not get calls until we decide to replace it. We will be successful more often and for longer periods with this strategy than with the first. Finally, we can get rid of the phone, or, we can remove ourselves from any proximity to a phone. This has the highest probability of success.

Similar general strategies can be generated for resisting the temptation to watch TV when we have other work to do. These include avoiding the TV room or placing the TV in an out-of-the-way place, getting rid of it, or removing ourselves temporarily to some environment which has no TV.

Behavioral modification can suggest a number of strategies for dealing with the environmental influences on eating behavior, just as it can for eliminating the influence of the telephone or TV set. It can also show us how to improve our self-control when we have to "guts it out," and even how to make new behavior more rewarding to us than our old habits. I will describe all of these techniques fully because they can work. Experimenters have applied these principles in the laboratory, and trained animals to perform amazing feats. In fact, it is not very difficult to set up a situation in which animals overeat or diet because the experimenter can exert very great control over an animal's environment. On the one hand, animals, like humans, tend to overeat on freely available fatty, sweetened, foods and get fat unless they can also be made to increase their activity. On the other hand, the experimenter can withhold food, make food difficult to get to, punish eating, or make a noneating response even more pleasurable than eating itself. And the animals will lose weight. Some of the same principles are used at "fat farms" to help people lose weight.

We know behavior modification principles work when we have strong control over an animal's or persons's environment. *Strong control* is the key phrase in this statement. Behavioral principles can't work if they are not used, and unless we want to live forever on a fat farm, *no one except ourselves controls the environment in which we eat. No one will impose on us the environmental changes that will force us to eat right, or get active, and be the thin people we say we want to be.*

Thus, in contrast with the experimental laboratory or the fat farm where someone else controls the setting and the rewards for learning, we have to take it upon ourselves to set up the best possible environment if we are serious about reaching our objectives. And we have to practice the behaviors I am going to describe *on our own initiative* if we want to see any changes. Our research has shown that just one change in eating behavior and one change in your thought processes, which I discuss later in this chapter, can predict weight management success.

With respect to eating behavior, people who change just one eating habit associated with poor nutrition or overeating, and who with absolute consistency maintain that *one* change over a period of several months, lose almost exactly twice the weight as others who flirt with different behavioral strategies and never make even one change permanent.

When you first start to make changes, you may wish to implement the behavioral strategy that seems easiest. Do that for one to two weeks. Then, after you've had a chance to evaluate the others that I suggest, pick the one that seems most appropriate for your particular eating problem. Occasionally, people stick with the same fervor to as many as two important stragegies, but, in my experience, two significant changes are about all anyone needs, or can be so consistent in using.

1. *Write down what you eat.* For one to two weeks, this strategy usually proves to be easiest to implement and the best one with which to begin. An eating record makes you aware of your eating behavior and helps you maintain your resolve—to "guts it out"— during the early period when you are making other important changes. Simply record what you eat, the type of food and quantity, either before, during, or after each meal. If you wait until evening to do an entire day, you may be inaccurate, and the strategy will not give you the control over your behavior as it does when you do it with each meal.

To get a feeling for this relatively easy change in your behavior, do it as I recommend during my Seven-Day Plan. If you find it especially helpful, keep it up throughout the dieting period.

2. *Keep all highly caloric foods that tempt you to overeat out of the house while dieting.* You will not have to do this after you've reached goal weight and gotten active, but: *the single most effective weight loss strategy* in my experience is to avoid temptation. In my telephone or TV examples, we cannot hear or see one if none is present. If the high calorie foods are nowhere around, we do not have to struggle to *resist* temptation. Don't put the food you overeat anywhere within walking distance. If you are like most people, myself included, if certain foods are freely available, the odds are you will ultimately

eat them to excess. This happens because sooner or later they manage to pop up right in front of our noses. We may see someone else eating them, or other family members may urge us to have a taste because they feel we are doing so well and deserve a reward. They use the phrase, "A little bit won't hurt." Not much.

I, like many overweight people with a large appetite for certain highly caloric foods, know very well the outcome when such foods are freely available in my environment. I have three weaknesses when it comes to such foods. I can easily eat one-half pound of chocolate, nut-covered toffee, or half a dozen old-fashioned style donuts, or a quart of rich ice cream at a single sitting. I still do it occasionally and I don't gain weight because I'm so active. But, I don't want to eat such large quantities of high fat, sugar foods as a general rule. So, except on rare occasions they stay out of the house. Because I need about 3000 calories a day to maintain my weight, I do need some concentrated calories. Dried fruit has become my substitute for ice cream, donuts, and candy.

To keep your food nemeses out of the house requires some negotiation with your family. You need to convince them of its value on a temporary basis for your health. Then, you might want to convince them of the value of trying to eat more nutritiously themselves. If they don't wish to change, you have to help them discover a way of satisfying their high calorie food appetites that won't endanger you, such as eating their fatty foods and desserts at meals taken away from home. Finally, you have to think of ways of repaying them for any collaboration they give you in making these changes.

Many people who work with me don't feel comfortable about imposing this home environment change on their families. Sometimes a mate or child will say, "Why do *I* have to be on a diet because *you* are trying to lose weight?" Most of the time, families will collaborate, at least on a temporary basis, once they understand how important this one change can be. They are usually more willing to collaborate when they see that *you* really mean business for once. Sometimes it takes a few weeks for them to be convinced of your motivation because they may have seen you engineer your own failure many times before. They know you have conflicting desires— you want to lose weight, but you still want to eat the foods that may be helping you stay fat. They know from past experience that the latter motivation finally wins out. *You* (not they) may buy or bake the high calorie foods and then eat them, even if you say you are buying such foods for them. Why should they change or be inconvenienced if you aren't serious and won't follow through yourself?

Most families want to help the overweight member lose weight. They soon begin to see how much better you look and feel and they begin to reap benefits themselves. When you are happier with yourself, you tend to be happier in your relationship with others.

But, if for some reason you cannot implement this very effective change strategy, here is second best:

3. *Repackage all high calorie foods in opaque containers or wrappers and put some sort of marking on them that clearly indicates they don't belong to you.* Some small file or address labels with the names of other people in the family will work well for this purpose. When you buy high calorie foods, buy exactly enough for the other members of the family, none for yourself, and rewrap them.

It may prove impossible to avoid seeing others eat the foods that tempt you. The best strategy is to leave the room when this occurs. One successful loser bought himself an electronic chess game. Every evening when the other members of his family dug into their high calorie desserts, he went out of the room and became absorbed in his chess game.

Here is a list of other helpful strategies. Try them and evaluate their effect on your eating behavior. Then stick with at least one with the tenacity of a bulldog. You will see the difference it can make.

4. *Do your food shopping from a list.*

5. *Plan several days' menus in advance.*

6. *Prepare only the quantity of food you plan to eat.*

7. *Do not serve meals family style (do not place full serving dishes on the dining table).*

8. *Let other people go out to the kitchen to serve themselves seconds.*

9. *Clear dishes directly into the garbage.*

Learning Alternate Behavior

All of the above strategies are designed either to get rid of certain foods from your environment or to limit quantities. This may

mean that eating behavior is going to be eliminated at times in which
it has been the most important and satisfying thing you do. By
stopping your eating behavior, you create a vacuum—you must put
something in its place that can come to give you the satisfaction
eating once did. Arrange to have some other activity readily available, as my chess playing patient did. Many people start activities
such as sewing, knitting, household repair chores, games, or paint-
ing, and set up an environment that makes it easy to become
involved with these activities when they might ordinarily have done
some unnecessary eating. This means leaving the materials for these
activities in plain sight and easily available. Sometimes these substitute activities come to yield as much intrinsic satisfaction as eating.
Late afternoon eaters and drinkers find that some sort of physical
activity results in even greater pleasure than eating, once it becomes
part of their lives. I strongly encourage you to follow their lead in
substituting activity for late afternoon eating. Sometimes, however,
the behavior you choose to substitute for eating never comes to feel
as good. You can still be successful in changing your behavior if
you set up some special schemes for rewarding yourself every time
you exhibit your desirable substitute behavior, and every time you
resist eating. You can supply your own positive reinforcement.

Supplying Positive Reinforcement

Most fat people concentrate on their weaknesses when it comes
to food. Their failures in weight management loom much larger in
their minds than their successes. The most important change you
can make in this regard is to consciously reflect upon—talk to yourself about—every single successful change in your behavior no
matter how small. As you engage my program you will begin each
day, of course, with that first minute of stretching when you get up
in the morning. Keep up the self-reinforcement talk when you eat
exactly the breakfast you have planned and pack that piece of fruit
to take with you to work. In this way, you incorporate both an eating and activity change in your life within moments after getting
up each morning.

During the rest of the day, opportunities for getting and giving
yourself positive reinforcement occur when you make your weight
management program obvious to others. Talk about what you are

doing and how you feel about it whenever it seems appropriate. Keep symbols of your changes in plain sight. Simple markers such as an apple on your desk, or putting this book out in a highly visible position, serve to keep your intentions salient. This will stimulate you to keep up a dialogue with yourself that reinforces every change you make. Others will note the presence of an apple or the book and ask questions, as they will about your pedometer. Talking to others about your program and your successes increases your commitment and resolve. Making changes becomes increasingly easier day by day.

Some other rewards to help you maintain your changed behaviors include:

1. Posting a weight graph showing your weekly (or daily if you prefer) weight.

2. Posting *thin* pictures of yourself if you have them, or a thin picture of the ideal toward which you are working in a conspicuous place.

3. Deposit a certain sum of money to a savings account for the successful completion of your behavior change strategy each day. I think you will do better if you reward yourself for behavior rather than weight loss. This is a particularly good strategy to increase your activity behavior. If you deposit a dollar for every mile walked you will soon have enough to buy the new clothes you are going to need. Put another dollar in for each day you stick with the Seven-Day Plan. You deserve a good new wardrobe.

4. Use symbols of physical activity to represent your new lifestyle. This takes your attention away from food and refocuses it on the new behaviors that will make you feel good. As with the apple, or copy of this book on your desk, put your walking shoes in a conspicuous place rather than in your closet. If you decide to use a walking stick, leave it out in plain sight. Buy some books on walking, yoga, or other physical activities and place them on tables in different rooms. Each time you lay your eyes on them, you can give yourself a quick pat on the back for all the changes you are making. A visible token of the new you in every room of the house will stimulate you to keep up the good work, keep your eating under control, and remind you to keep up the positive dialogue with yourself.

Self-Control Techniques

Changing the act of eating itself might help you control your overall intake. If you happen to be a fast eater, especially if you are aware of eating your problem foods in a comparatively more excited, higher drive state, you may find it worthwhile to cultivate a slower pace.

Because it is almost as difficult to change the physical act of eating as it is to change the way you place your feet when walking, I never insist that fast eaters learn to change. Even among successful weight losers, very few in my experience indicate that they were successful in learning to become slow eaters. They attribute their success to other factors—usually their activity level, keeping junk foods out of the house, and menu planning.

But since fast eating is generally not as satisfying or as good for your digestive processes as slow eating, here is a way to slow down. Use one or more of the steps. The more you use the more likely you are to succeed.

1. Start the meal by sitting quietly for at least one full minute. Relax to get rid of any high tension state you may have brought to the dining table. Slowly saying "Grace" proves to be an excellent beginning for many people.

2. If you are with a group of people, be the last person to start eating.

3. As you start to eat, focus on the taste of each mouthful. Doing the tasting experiment with herbs during my Seven-Day Plan will give you some practice in becoming aware of food flavors.

4. Choose a slow eating model if you are in a group. Inconspicuously, pace your eating along with that other person.

5. Stop at least once about mid-way through the meal for a minute and rest.

6. Do not put any food on your fork or take a bite of sandwich until you have completely chewed and swallowed each mouthful. *Watch that fork!* It seems to have a life of its own. Fast eaters fill it immediately after placing its contents in their mouths. This is a particularly hard behavior to change. You may want to put your fork down after each bite, or carefully let it touch your plate, *empty,* until you swallow.

7. If you are not using a slow eating model to follow, *be the last*

at the table to finish. If you have eaten faster than the slowest person, this means intentionally saving a bit of food until everyone has finished.

8. To be successful in slowing your eating requires continual, conscious effort. You are taking an activity that is usually automatic—like driving or walking—and forcing yourself to attend to its components. This can become very uncomfortable and frustrating. To avoid failure, keep relaxed, don't kick yourself when you forget to stick to your plan, and keep rewarding yourself for every minute of success.

9. Don't declare "From now on I am going to eat slowly." Pick *one* meal with which to experiment and see how slow eating feels. Then decide if you want to do it again. Next, decide if you want to practice slow eating for one meal each day. In this unpressured way, the change may sneak up on you without the feeling of effort and frustration that most people experience when they try to slow down without a graduated plan.

Dealing with Other People

For some dieters, the support of family and friends can be critical. You are most likely to get their support when they realize you are serious, that losing weight is a high priority item in your life, and when they understand why you are doing each thing in your program. They will maintain their support and change their behavior as long as you repay them, thank them, or otherwise reciprocate for their help. You don't have to be gushy or artificial about expressing your appreciation. A simple thanks for any specific helpful act is plenty. Several weeks down the line (when they least expect it) an announcement of how well you are doing and how much you appreciate their overall help will be very reinforcing and make them feel good. This kind of thanks is a compliment to them as a person, rather than for a particular act.

Before someone can be helpful to you, however, they have to know what is helpful and what isn't. Sometimes it is possible to specify in advance what these things are and will be, and consistency in offering support in a particular way may always prove to be helpful. But we are changeable beings. Some days a simple question like, "How are you doing with your program?" is welcome, but on other days, the same question can be irritating. Our response may be dictated by a number of other events which affect our mood and have nothing much to do with the success of our program. When this happens, it's helpful to be aware of the things that are irritating us. We can indicate to our family and friends that while we know they have good intentions, pursuing the topic is not going to be helpful at this particular time.

Eating out with friends or being a dinner guest often poses some special problems. We feel uncomfortable if we hurt another's feelings when they offer us a high calorie dish, or when they invite us for a snack and coffee break. Most of the time we are simply imagining their reactions. They would not be in the least offended by a "no thanks" or a "no thanks" with a small explanation. I solved the problem by announcing my new Four-S diet, and it never once failed in preventing another person from urging me to eat. You may find a quick reference to your new diet when high calorie foods are offered, or an advance warning when invited out—to suffice. "Will you have some chocolate cake?" can be answered with "Would you be offended if I refused (or said 'no thanks')? I'm on my __th day of my __ day reducing plan, I can't deviate now." Frankly, you have no obligation to explain yourself, and that brief "Would you be offended" disarms almost everyone.

One of the better ways to get the support of friends and family is to get someone else to go on your program with you. In the case of your mate, you can both use similar diets, but you don't have to be physically active at the same time. However, if both mates take up an activity program, you have to help each other find time, and chances of mutual support increase. The same with diet, but be ready for the fact that men will usually lose faster than women. The companionship of a friend at your job site can be helpful. You need to decide whether you want to emphasize a competitive or collaborative approach. I think collaboration in changing behavior rather than competition in speed of weight loss is the better strategy. If you tie success to weight loss, one of you may be somewhat discouraged in a competition.

Dealing with Emotions

Many people turn to food when they are anxious, tense, bored, or angry. Sometimes these emotions seem to drive us to seek out food when we are not really hungry. At other times the presence of tension increases the speed of eating and the amount we consume at our regular meal times, usually dinner.

You have three options in dealing with the eating-emotions relationship.

1. Change the situations that elicit the emotional reaction.

2. Learn to change your emotional response to a given situation.

3. Learn to change your behavior in response to your emotions.

You may wish to emphasize one of these three options in making changes, but you will find that a change in any one aspect has an impact on the others. Let's analyze some typical examples.

High drive states that lead to overeating can arise from stressful work settings, other tensions, personal relationships, or "big holes" in one's life. By big holes I mean absence of satisfaction from work, in personal relationships, or simply nothing to do for certain periods after work each day or on weekends.

Dealing directly with other people whose behavior elicits strong emotion requires a willingness to express your feelings and the ability to assert your legitimate rights and needs. For this you need confidence in your worth as a person, and often some practice in developing assertive skills. Many overweight people feel unworthy simply because they are fat. And many, because they are fat, feel that the only way they can continue to be liked or accepted is to "stomach" their feelings. Because they believe their acceptance in society or personal relationships is borderline at best, they don't dare to express negative emotions directly for fear of total rejection.

Fortunately, getting active and engaging in a working weight control program has that mysterious side effect which leads to increased independence and self-confidence. You don't even need to try, to obtain these benefits. But, you can speed up the process. You do not have to be "right or wrong" to state your feelings about behavior that disturbs you when your goal is to work things out with mutual satisfaction.

The first step is to become aware of what events elicit the emotions that ultimately result in overeating. Sometimes there can be a series or chain that culminates, several hours later, in a large eating episode. For example, you build up a reservoir of tension at work (and you may also be building a hidden hunger drive to go with it if you are skipping meals), you get home to some tasks or interactions with your family that cause anger or anxiety, and you stuff at dinner until you can't move. At each step of the way you can prevent the buildup of extra tension by letting off a little steam. Use this four-step process for making your first efforts to change:

1. Identify the events or the behaviors of other people that elicit negative emotions.

2. Get clear on how you would like them to be changed, so that you can state your wishes as explicitly as possible. If you cannot see your way clearly, then just be prepared to say so, but open the discussion.

3. Identify in yourself what aspect of your own behavior may be adding to your discomfort. Perhaps you are only a little annoyed with someone else, but doubly annoyed because you aren't pleased with your own response.

4. Get clear on how you want to change your own reactions to such situations.

Once you have gone through these four steps, role play the new and desired situation in your mind—practice the way you will deal with the situation when it next occurs. Some people take time to write out their scenario. It is helpful to discuss each element in your plan—even rehearse it—with a friend.

When you start dealing directly with situations that cause negative emotions, you may find that your reactions to that situation begin to change in the process. You will take pride in the fact that you have expressed yourself and you will no longer feel helpless about your power to change the way you are being treated.

If you decide not to make a special effort to change a bad situation, or if change is impossible, then your second option is to learn to modify your reactions themselves. If tension is a factor, learning to let loose and relax can become one of the most useful skills in your behavioral repertoire. Some people gain considerable release from tension by finding a new phrase that they repeat to themselves when they feel tension rising. Something like, "Whoa," or "Wait a minute, slow down," followed by a few deep breaths. A common physical site for tension lies in the neck and shoulders. When you feel tension in that area of your body, take a short time out, turn your head slowly from side to side, rotate your shoulders forward and back and feel some of the tension subside. A popular book which has helped many people learn the relaxation response is a book by that title by H. Benson.* A five-minute time-out for yoga, and a few exercises of your choice from chapters five and thirteen may prove helpful. If possible, leave the area in which you are experiencing your tension and go to a different location. That spot will soon begin to act as a special stimulus area for the relaxation response. Just sitting quietly for five minutes with eyes closed in such a special spot can be helpful. If, during this time, you want to empty your mind from an annoying obsessive thought, focus it on some simple task such as counting slowly backwards from ninety-nine to zero. If necessary, do it three times. When your mind wanders as it may, just bring it back to the nearest digit you recall before you were distracted and continue counting down. It takes about five minutes to do this three times and you will experience considerable relief from negative feelings by the time you finish.

A social sport at the end of the afternoon may release tension that leads to overeating later that night. This is a good time for a tennis or racquet ball game. I find that the best antidote for negative emotion lies in activities such as walking, jogging, or swimming for that forty-five-minute period I keep speaking about. The rhythmic aspect of these activities acts like the chanting of a mantra in meditation. In addition, these activities burn a lot of calories. I think you will find an overall improvement in your mood and very likely a change in your response to many situations that previously made you feel tense or anxious once you get that forty-five minutes a day into your activity program.

When implementing one or both of the above options does not seem to work, your final resort is to find a substitute for eating when negative emotions seem to drive you in that direction. The technique is similar in some respects to what I have just finished describing. To begin with, once again you must realize that you are the one responsible for initiating and practicing any new response you wish to acquire when you decide to eliminate emotional eating. You must decide which substitute response or set of responses you will use. It may take weeks of practice for you to see a significant change. Of course, I recommend some sort of physical activity as a replacement for eating. A walk, or some stretching, will alleviate

---

*Benson, H. *The Relaxation Response*. New York: Morrow, 1975.

tension and give you a feeling of being in control. If you would ordinarily eat for five, ten, or fifteen minutes, walk or do some yoga instead for exactly that period of time. You can set a timer for some predetermined period—engage in your substitute activity—and then reconsider whether you still want to eat. A hot shower is also an excellent substitute. If you are bursting with anger, beat on a pillow or go into a closet and scream. Finally, if you cannot defeat the nibbles, you are still relatively safe if you have rid your environment of high calorie foods and force yourself to eat at least one large carrot and a whole grapefruit before you get into the car to drive to the candy store or ice cream parlor. You can always eat your fill of fresh fruits and vegetables.

Changing Your Cognitive Environment

"I don't have any willpower when it comes to food." That statement is among the most frequent self-evaluative statements fat people make about themselves. If this is the sort of thing you say to yourself, you can probably look back on innumerable times when your resistance has broken down as proof of its validity. But you may not realize how that self-description predicts, even aids, future failure. It's a vicious cycle. Every time you overeat, you kick yourself and think you have no willpower. Then, just saying that kind of thing to yourself creates a hopeless frame of mind. It can prevent you from taking steps to change both your behavior and the self-talk that reflect your negative attitude.

We all *can* change our behavior and our self-evaluation. But we usually make the mistake of aiming too high. We want perfection immediately. We don't realize that it takes a reasonable plan of action and practice. Remember, mountain climbers don't start with Mount Everest. They go into a long period of training; conquering smaller mountains gives them the strength and wisdom to tackle the biggies.

Let's accept one fact at the onset. If we like high calorie foods and can eat monstrous quantities, it is surely unreasonable to expect that we will ever grow to hate them and *never want* to eat them again. This reversal has happened to a few people but it is extremely rare. Usually, we simply learn how to control our behavior and begin to say to ourselves the things that help us carry out our control. Once we see that learning new behavior protects us from overeating, we feel confident and say we have all the willpower we need to be the kind of person we want to be. Then we can make a decision to eat, even overeat on occasion, knowing that we can stop and prevent future occurrences whenever we want to. Naturally, becoming active enough to burn several hundred calories every day removes the need to exercise perfect restraint. Furthermore, when we *can* eat more every day without getting fat, the tension that accompanies the need to watch food intake like a hawk is lessened. Often, the lessening of tension reduces the danger of a binge. We also gain confidence in the knowledge that an occasional bash does not make an active person fat.

In order to change our cognitive environment from negative to positive, we build on the self-reinforcement technique I discussed earlier in the chapter. Every time we carry out a new behavior no matter how small, it's a step in the right direction and illustrates our power to change. It's a rule! Keep your successes up front in your awareness. It helps to review your successes each day, before you go to sleep at night.

You can, in addition, develop a plan for the specific purpose of giving you a sense of willpower. It works this way. If you analyze any given situation in which you overeat you will see that the final act of overeating has been preceded by a series or chain of earlier events. These include thoughts, emotions, and behaviors that take place in certain settings. Before you eat your tenth cookie you have to eat your ninth. Before you have your first, they must be present in your environment. In order to be present and within reaching distance, you must move near them, or someone must bring them to you. In the very first place they had to be purchased or baked.

Let's take a look at the thoughts that may occur along the way to the tenth cookie. If you eat them at home, you may permit their presence because you think they should be available for the rest of your family. That is obviously self-deception. It's you that's eating them and not the rest of your family. Before you ate the first cookie, you thought to yourself or someone said to you, "Just one won't hurt." But after the third cookie, perhaps, you said "The hell with it. I've blown it for the day, so I may as well polish them off and start dieting again tomorrow."

Let's take a look at some feelings. When the thought of eating a cookie hits you, you may have felt a bit of tension, some conflict. Should you or shouldn't you? As you had your first bite, perhaps, you felt guilty already. Perhaps, like many, many fat people, you felt some excitement or anxiety—a rising drive state. Perhaps as a result of these feelings you began to eat faster. Soon you were hardly tasting, you were chewing and swallowing so fast. That's when all restraint left you and you gave up completely. And you downed the rest of the cookies in that typical mixed state of the overeater— loving and hating every bite simultaneously.

You can practice getting control—developing willpower—at every stage of the way along this path. But the longer you wait to interrupt the chain, the harder it gets. Here are two more rules:

1. The earlier the chain is interrupted, the easier it is to succeed in getting control of it.

2. A practiced alternative response ready at every stage increases your chances of control if, somehow, early steps are skipped. This may happen, for example, when someone presents you with your favorite chocolate cake at a surprise birthday party or wedding anniversary.

Here is a summary of a typical chain of events that can lead to undesirable overeating of a high calorie food. I use chocolate chip cookies as an example but the process can be generalized to other foods and situations. As I discuss each link in the chain, I suggest which of the strategies are best suited to making changes, together with the thoughts you can attach to your actions as you create a positive cognitive environment.

Chocolate chip cookies purchased or baked The single most effective strategy: don't buy or bake them. If *you* do the buying or baking, ask yourself why? Isn't it true that, regardless of your rationale, *you* end up eating them? This reflects the conflict of opposing motivations. Shop from a list, or let someone else do the shopping. Let others in your family buy their own sweets, or bake them for themselves, and make sure that only enough for the other members of the family are present in the environment. If you do the shopping, buy good substitute foods to satisfy your hunger, and if it's baking, find a substitute activity for baking. Each time you successfully complete a shopping trip without purchasing high calorie foods and each time you find something satisfying to do instead of cookie making, pat yourself on the back for your success.

These are the first and best steps you can take to control an eating problem. And remember, this much restraint is only temporary.

Chocolate chip cookies in the house   Use opaque wrappers and a label with the names of people who can include them in their diet. Stare at the packages—*they belong to someone else.* Let the other family members store them and retrieve them when they're going to eat some. Each successful avoidance on your part is a demonstration of your willpower.

Cookies in sight   Put them away yourself, or if others are eating them, go to another room. Or, ask others to eat some place else. Have a substitute activity ready if the eating urge strikes. Engage it immediately—don't wait a single second.

If you wish to learn to resist food right in front of your nose, this too can be done. It's risky, however, and very few people who enjoy sweets ever become perfect in doing it. Practicing the behavior I suggest can be a help, however, even if it works only a certain percentage of the time.

Set up a special practice session when your desire to eat cookies is low. It's good to have a friend around the first time. Explain that you want to learn to be in the presence of a food that tempts you and not eat it. Set the cookies out in plain sight and leave them there. If you experience no urge to eat them, reflect on your feelings—it *is* possible to be around cookies without eating them. Rehearse thoughts like, "I *used* to eat cookies every time I got near one," and "I can be around such stuff and not eat."

If an urge arises in a practice situation, it will probably be less intense than usual and easy to resist. Think of how you used to give in and how much weight you gained after a binge. Now you are not giving in.

Put the cookies away. Repeat this practice session several times on different days.

Cookies within reach   Move out of reach, or ask others to remove the food. You can continue your practice of resisting food when in its presence by reaching and stopping yourself. Think, "I can do anything I want about these cookies. I can eat or not. I'm not going to eat now." Do it again and again. Say it to yourself aloud. Do it until the desire to pick one up gets less and less, or disappears completely.

Cookie in hand   Pick up a cookie. Put it back. Think, "I've changed my mind. I don't believe I'll have any until I reach my weight goal. Then I'll see if I want one."

Three helpful strategies in dealing with undesirable food in the hand are: throwing it away, giving it away, and messing it up.

By and large, fat people hurt inside when they throw food away. Some feel it's a sin. They have to function as garbage pails. Cleaning up everyone's leftovers, or forcing down the last bit of cake and cookies in the box, is a well-established habit. The acts have been performed hundreds of times. But throwing something out? Never.

With practice, you can get over the discomfort associated with throwing food away. Buy a whole box of cookies—the more expensive the better. One by one, throw them away. Reflect on your feelings. If you are like most fat people, you can hardly force yourself to do this. Most fat people never fully appreciate how much they love these foods. It actually tears their hearts out to throw something like this away. They then realize that if such foods are around, they will ultimately eat them unless they can change their reactions to the sight of the food in a garbage pail.

If you persist and actually throw all the cookies away, and if you keep doing it—possibly hundreds of times—the act of throwing undesirable food away can become as easy and automatic as eating it. If you want that power to resist, use every opportunity to throw leftovers or undesirable food away if it gets into your presence. You can elect yourself to do the cleaning up after dinner. Have someone watch and assist you getting unwanted leftovers into the garbage pail. Some people say things to themselves like, "Here, garbage pail—*you* get fat, not I."

Practice giving food away. This is most helpful after a party when you have decided to include potentially dangerous food in the menu. This is what I do after we have some high calorie desserts that I might gorge on in the future. I am not good at resisting, and I don't want to become perfect at it. So, I just give such foods away to my guests. Practice this giveaway with the last few cookies in your practice session by giving them to your friend to take home. If your friend is on the program with you, he or she can throw them away and get some good practice.

Messing up food can help you develop a distaste for it. I have helped several people with exceedingly strong drives for candy and cola (two foods I think you can permanently eliminate without harm to your health or asthetic sensibilities) get rid of their urges by mixing these foods with vinegar, pepper, dirt, and ashes. If you stare at them and smell them a few times in this condition and develop a clear mental picture of the situation, you may never want to eat those foods again, or your aversion may last at least throughout the period you wish to diet.

I don't like the "mess-it-up" strategy. I use it only in extreme cases. I hate to mess up the high calorie foods I like best and by using avoidance and substitution strategies I can still eat them on occasion with great enjoyment and without doing it to excess. However, some of my patients carry small plastic packages of salt, pepper, and mustard in their purses. If they are ever tempted to eat food not in their menu plan, they whip out their defensive weapons and mess up their pie in public.

Cookies eaten   It won't help to kick yourself. Shame, guilt, and self-punishment haven't worked in the past and they won't work now. Just because you like cookies doesn't make you a lousy person. You simply prefer the gratification of eating them to the reward of losing weight. Or, perhaps, you want to give increased activity itself a try, and continue eating the way you like, even if it takes longer. When you decide to include a temporary diet in your plans, go back to step one and begin again.

Stop Trying

At the beginning of this chapter I said that one behavioral and one cognitive factor seem to be associated with weight management success. The behavioral factor is seen in the absolutely consistent use of usually one and occasionally two strategies to change the environment or one's own eating behavior while dieting. The cognitive factor is reflected in the use of the word "try." People who use the word "try" in statements such as, "I'm trying to walk more," or "I'm trying to diet" are the ones who fail. These are the persons who do not want to *do* the things that make weight loss possible, even easy. You do not need to "try" to walk. You already *know* how. You may have to negotiate time to do it, but when a person uses that word "try" when it comes to walking, I know he or she is not strongly motivated to do the most important thing necessary for permanent weight control: get active.

The same goes for dieting. "I'm trying to diet." Or, "I'm trying to eat more nutritiously," tells me that that person's mind is prepared for failure. You already know what to do to control your intake—that's what this chapter is about. *Do*—don't try!

I believe this cognitive change is fundamental to the consistent use of any behavioral change strategy. Are you going to be a "doer" or a "tryer?" Think about it and then keep repeating to yourself the kind of person you are—but only if you do decide to *do*, not try.

12

DEALING WITH SLOW METABOLISM

"I eat like a bird. I have friends who eat twice as much as I do and they stay skinny while I can't lose weight. All I need to do is look at food and I get fat."

I believe you. Many people who try to lose weight by cutting back on caloric intake and do not become active have difficulty with standard reducing diets. There are two reasons for this.

1. There is considerable variability in basal metabolism. Given two persons of the same sex, age, and lifestyle, one may *lose* weight on 2300 calories, another *gain* on 1700. Admittedly, these would be people somewhat at the extremes of metabolic requirements, but it does occur.

2. Metabolic reaction to caloric restriction varies. In one case, metabolism may slow as little as 10 percent in response to a low calorie diet, but in another, it may slow 45 percent.

Recent research has just barely opened the door to what may finally result in an understanding of all the biochemical processes involved in these metabolic differences.

To begin with, we can infer that genetic influences on biochemical processes exist in humans on the basis of family history. We stop at the level of inference because it is difficult to separate such influences from eating and activity habits transmitted from parents to children. With some strains of animals, however, we can clearly determine the genetic basis and can breed for fatness or thinness. A great deal of research is focused on investigating differences in cell function, hormone levels, and enzymes in fat and thin individuals, using both animals and humans as subjects. Not everything that we discover in laboratory work with animals will be true of humans, of course, but it can show us where to look.

At this early point in the research on biochemical differences between the obese and nonobese, we can conclude that many factors, each alone, or acting together with others, can predispose a person to obesity and difficulties in losing weight.

1. Body cells in the obese may do their work, rebuilding themselves, regenerating, getting energy and nutrients in and wastes out, with much greater efficiency. The cells of thin people may be wasteful of energy. This is suggested by the fact that more heat is given off by the fat cells of the thin, than by the fat cells of the obese. Similarly, much energy, possibly 25 to 50 percent of our basal metabolic needs, is used to maintain a certain chemical balance between body cells and the surrounding fluids. Each of us has billions and billions of cells in our bodies working to keep sodium at a relatively lower internal concentration compared with the surrounding fluid, while letting potassium in. Cells of the obese seem to do this work much more efficiently, that is, using less energy.

2. Animals and humans possess a small amount of a very active kind of fat tissue called brown fat. It burns calories at many times the rate of ordinary fat. The naturally thin may have relatively more of this kind of fat or be able to generate more of it in response to an increased caloric intake. This would help keep them thin.

3. There can be as much as a fivefold variation in the levels of hormones and enzymes involved in energy storage and utilization. A person whose body produces a large quantity of enzymes that convert the energy in food to fat for storage, but few that reconvert it back from storage to utilization will be predisposed to obesity. The same with the many hormones associated with the use of energy. Slight variations in one direction or another in insulin, thyroid, catecholamines, and endorphins (there may be many others) can predispose us to obesity. These deviations can effect our appetite as well as the efficiency with which our bodies accomplish their physiological functions.

4. Some of these physiological differences may be caused not by genetic influences but by our lifestyles. Through overeating and underactivity our bodies develop their full potential to produce the hormones and enzymes needed for fat storage. It's true that the

body tries to waste some calories when we begin to overeat, but if we stay inactive and keep on overeating, we help, possibly even *force*, the obesity producing mechanisms win out and become stabilized. Then as I explained in chapter three, by going to the other extreme, with repeated low calorie dieting, we encourage yet other mechanisms to begin working to protect our already highly developed fat storage capacity. When we convert to moderate eating and an active lifestyle, we encourage opposite mechanisms. Enzymes and hormone levels are changed in ways to facilitate adaptation to a more active life. Much more research is needed to determine the extent to which our lifestyle produces such changes, and how long it takes to make them.

5. Certain drugs in common use, such as tranquilizers, some hormones, and blood pressure medications slow metabolism, foster weight gain, and hinder weight loss. Be sure to discuss whatever medications you are taking with your physician. If you discover that you are using some medication that slows metabolism or encourages fat storage, you should ask for frequent checkups— perhaps monthly—to determine whether alterations in the dosage are necessary as you lose weight and get fit. *Never discontinue prescribed medications without your doctor's advice.* Abrupt changes or discontinuation can be extremely dangerous. As soon as your physician sees that you are serious and committed to your new lifestyle, *and that he can trust you to continue your health enhancing behaviors, then he can feel free to reduce or eliminate medication that may previously have been necessary* (even though weight gain has been an unfortunate side effect).

Do You Have Slow Metabolism?

There is a very simple answer to this question. No. Not if you average one and one-half to two pounds a week of weight loss on the approximately 1200 calories I suggest in my Double Your Fat Loss Diet and forty-five minutes a day of walking. You will lose more than that the first two weeks—some people lose three to four times that much (remember, it's mostly water)—and then settle into a fairly stable pattern. You may experience an occasional plateau, even a few pounds up after a high sodium meal or before a menstrual period, but with no serious metabolic deviation, you should

average, over time, between one and one-half and two pounds a
week beginning about week three.

Unless you have been keeping strictly to a relatively low calorie
diet for a long period of time, or have repeatedly dieted at 1000
calories or less, the probability that you have a metabolic deviation
that's worth getting concerned about is quite low, especially if you
are less than fifty pounds overweight. At more than fifty pounds
overweight, with continual dieting or repeated low calorie diets, the
probability of slow metabolism increases. However, at the onset of
your weight loss program there is no need to keep the very extensive records necessary to evaluate your metabolism. Just follow my
recommendations and see what happens. If your average loss is less
than expected, then it's time to get serious about your metabolic
rate and take what special steps you can to raise it or compensate.

Evaluating Your Own Metabolism

The tests for metabolic rate usually done in the physician's office
are incomplete and possibly inaccurate. It takes sophisticated
equipment and repeated measurements under well-controlled conditions to obtain a reliable evaluation.

Unless a metabolic laboratory is available, and you want to invest
considerably money, the next best approach to determine whether
your caloric needs are average, above, or below, is to keep an accurate eating and weight record. These can be supplemented by an
activity record, just to see if intake, expenditure, and weight have
the predicted relationship. I describe how to keep an activity record
at the end of this chapter. It's optional and for many reasons, not
as likely to be as accurate as your eating record. An eating record
and your weight over a long period of time are all you need.

Before you begin I must correct a misconception you may have
about what is necessary to determine your true "baseline" eating
behavior and the amount of time and effort involved in the process
of determining your caloric needs. Some commercial programs and
weight loss manuals suggest that you keep an eating diary for one
week to determine your usual eating habits and the number of calories it takes to maintain your weight. This is not adequate for at
least two reasons. You are likely to alter your eating habits when
you first monitor them, but even if you didn't, the body regulates

its intake-expenditure balance over extremely long periods of time. It will take several weeks of conscientious measurement to obtain a reasonably adequate self-evaluation. Fortunately, it can be done while dieting, as well as during a period when you are maintaining a stable weight. Thus, this metabolic self-evaluation can be used simultaneously as a weight loss strategy. As you do it, you will learn to predict your weight loss averaged over time and have the satisfaction of learning about your bodily processes and your ability to control them.

Equipment   You need a scale to weigh your food, a measuring cup and spoons, a reliable scale to weigh yourself, a complete calorie counter, a notebook to record your food intake and body weight on a daily basis, and a great deal of patience.

Procedure   Weigh yourself each morning after urination. If you use a balance beam scale, one weighing is enough. If you use a standard bathroom scale, get on and off three times, and take the average. Stand the same way on the scale at every weighing.

Keep absolutely accurate eating records by weighing and measuring everything. Start week three of your diet after your large initial water loss. Record the calories and every single bit of food and drink. Although your calorie counters will not be perfectly accurate because the same amount of food can vary in calorie content (depending on a number of factors, such as time of year for fruits and vegetables, marbling in meats) if you are careful over a four week period, you can feel reasonably certain that you are within 10 percent of your actual intake. On the basis of this record and your rate of weight loss, you can estimate your body's caloric deficit while dieting and make a good guess as to the amount you will be able to eat when you reach your goal.

Starting at week three, every pound of weight loss represents approximately a 3500-calorie deficit in your intake. Over a twenty-eight-day period, total up the calories you have eaten from your eating record. Then total the calories represented in your weight loss. Divide each by twenty-eight.

If you are a woman and have been following my suggestions, you should have an average intake of approximately 1200 calories (a man can be as high as 1800 calories). If you have a reasonably normal metabolic rate and have faithfully gotten in your forty-five minutes a day of brisk walking, you should have lost six to eight pounds in these four weeks. A six-pound loss represents a 21,000-calorie deficit, or 750 calories a day below the average person's weight maintenance level. It suggests that once you finish dieting, you will be able to eat at least 1950 calories a day if you are a woman, provided you stay active. You will be able to eat proportionately more if you are a man.

Suppose you deviate from these predictions. What would still be considered normal? While the average woman in her twenties weighing 128 pounds and doing the activities I suggest would need around 2000 calories to maintain her weight (a man of 154 pounds, 2700), a deviation of 400 calories in either direction does not imply gross metabolic disturbance. Thus, if you have lost only four pounds in four weeks, it means your actual expenditure averaged only 1700 calories if you are a woman eating 1200 calories, or about 2300 if you are a man on an 1800-calorie intake. You should still feel encouraged to know that you can eat at least that much and not gain weight once you reach your goal and keep your activity level up.

Calculating Caloric Needs After Dieting

Once you have reached your weight goal and stopped dieting, give your body at least two weeks to adjust to a higher food intake. Your weight will fluctuate, possibly as much as two pounds a day up or down and you may put a couple of pounds of water weight back on, so keep a weight record and determine that your average weight in the last three days of week two is about equal to that of the first three days. Then start keeping your eating diary and weight record again.

Table 3 contains the approximate average calorie needs of men and women in their twenties who add forty-five minutes of daily activity to an otherwise sedentary lifestyle. Since basal metabolism and the calorie needs of exercise are reduced with age in sedentary people, if you are over thirty years of age, adjust your needs downward by .5 percent per year (or 5 percent per decade).*

*Recent research shows that this commonly observed, age-related metabolic decline is caused largely by a decrease in muscle mass that occurs with a decline in activity levels as we grow older. By staying active and preserving your muscle mass with the program I recommend, you can prevent a slowing of your metabolic rate to a great extent. An active fifty-year-old person can burn as much as 10 percent more calories just sitting still, compared with a sedentary fifty-year-old who has lost muscle mass and replaced it with fat tissue.

TABLE 3

*Average Caloric Needs: Age 22 ***

BODY WEIGHT		
KG	POUNDS	CALORIC ALLOWANCE
MEN		
50	110	2200
55	121	2350
60	132	2500
65	143	2650
70	154	2800
75	165	2950
80	176	3050
85	187	3200
90	198	3350
95	209	3500
100	220	3700
WOMEN		
40	88	1550
45	99	1700
50	110	1800
55	121	1950
58	128	2000
60	132	2050
65	143	2200
70	154	2300

*These calculations assume that a person is at desirable weight and not obese. Obese individuals use fewer calories per pound of body weight. Thus, an obese sedentary woman of 200 pounds may need no more calories to maintain her weight than an active woman at 128 pounds desirable weight. Calorie requirements decrease with age about 5 percent per decade in sedentary people. A deviation of up to 400 calories in either direction from the average values listed is still considered to be within the normal range.

Dealing With Slower-than-Predicted Weight Loss

Unless you are demonstrably deficient in hormones that affect energy utilization, it is not wise to take any drug to speed up metabolism. If you do, it should always be under a knowledgeable physician's direction. Any drug that speeds up metabolism may cause the body to decrease its own production of that or related substances. The safest course of action is to change your behavior in such a way as to encourage your body to use its own resources.

My recommendations are based on the following facts:

1. Every time you eat, there may be a slight elevation in your metabolic rate (this may not occur or be quite small in very obese individuals).

2. This rise can be magnified by physical activity.

3. When you eat one large meal a day, most of the caloric intake must be converted for fat storage only to be slowly withdrawn over the next several hours. This keeps up your fat cells' ability to store fat.

4. Overweight individuals tend to be very efficient in their work. They are constantly saving steps.

Therefore, if you are not losing at least one pound a week,

1. Eat three regular meals of no more than 300 calories each. Add three snacks of 100 calories each. After each of the three regular meals, *walk for fifteen minutes.* This will be, for you, the best way to get in your forty-five minutes' worth of activity.

2. If you drink coffee or tea, which can slightly elevate your metabolic rate, drink one cup at breakfast and one at lunch time.

3. Drink plenty of water. Force yourself. Your body will have to work to get rid of it.

4. Avoid alcohol.

5. In addition to your walking, be sure to do the light weight lifting exercises I recommend, or upper body calisthenics, to build your muscle mass.

6. Move around at every opportunity. If you have a sitting job, spend five minutes an hour in some nonsitting activity such as stretching, stair climbing, or walking. Your increased productivity in the other fifty-five minutes will more than make up for the five-

minute break. Do all of your socializing while walking, not sitting. If you add five minutes of walking and stair climbing each hour in an eight-hour work day, you will burn approximately 200 more calories. This could make the difference you are looking for.

When to See Your Physician about Slow Metabolism

The activity program I recommend can compensate for as much as a 20 percent deviation on the slow side in your body metabolism. You must do it religiously and, as your condition improves, do it as briskly as is safe and comfortable to obtain the greatest benefit. If you find it difficult to lose weight on 1200 calories (1500–1800 for a man) be sure to maximize the metabolic benefits of the suggestions I have just made above. Consider also that each mile of walking is approximately equal to about 5 percent of a woman's daily caloric needs. *It is much better when possible to add an extra mile of walking to combat slow metabolism than it is to cut back another 100 calories in your diet.* Cutting back on eating may only slow you down some more.

However, if you are not able to lose a pound a week on the diet I recommend and have been faithfully adding forty-five minutes of walking daily (your pedometer must show five to six miles total a day to match the energy requirements in table 3) your metabolism is enough on the slow side to warrant professional supervision of your weight loss. Similarly, if a woman regains weight (instead of holding steady) while faithfully adhering to a daily activity program and eating 1700 calories, it merits professional evaluation.

Do not bother your doctor, however, unless you have an honest record averaging a 1200 calorie daily intake and a history of forty-five minutes of daily activity to go with little or no weight loss over a four-week period. It simply isn't worth your time and money to go through needless tests. The greatest danger is that by not keeping an honest record you will delude yourself and your doctor into thinking you have a metabolic problem where none exists. The simple remedy (to such a nonexisting problem) is to prescribe needless thyroid medication or appetite suppressants that contain stimulants. This "solution" may only make it more difficult to lose or maintain a lower weight later on. In fact, except for people who have fasted to lose a large amount of weight and then regained it, I find people who have used amphetamines about the hardest to help the second (or third, or fourth) time around.

Do not be impatient with the slowness of a one-pound-a-week weight loss. I talk with many women who go on and off 800-to 1000-calorie diets losing twelve pounds in a hurry only to regain a baker's dozen in an equal amount of time. Do not use such diets unless absolutely necessary, never without becoming active, and only under professional supervision.

Matching Energy Expenditure with Intake—the Activity Record

Caloric needs vary because we differ in basal metabolic requirements and because we differ in the amount of energy we use doing identical activities. Part of these differences is due to body composition as well as to biochemical variations. Two people of identical body size and weight will not have the same caloric needs if one has less fat mass and more lean mass than the other. Another part of the difference is due to body weight itself. It costs a heavier person more energy to walk than it does a light person. We also differ in the efficiency of our movements or the amount of needless tension in these movements. For example, agile, well-coordinated tennis players who anticipate where the ball is going, use considerably less energy than less-gifted or accomplished players. However, better players play at higher levels of intensity and expend more energy in a given period of time than novices.

For these reasons, as well as because it is an even greater bother than keeping an eating record, an activity diary based on standard energy expenditure charts calculated for the average person is likely to be much less accurate than an eating diary. Nevertheless, it is interesting to see how close you can come in making estimates of your eating and activity match your weight changes over an extended period.

Table 4 presents approximate energy requirements for various activities per kilogram of body weight. Study the directions for using it and the examples which follow.

TABLE 4

Approximate Energy Costs of Various Activities
for Persons of Average Weight *

ACTIVITY	KCAL / MIN KG	ACTIVITY	KCAL / MIN KG
Archery	0.065	Cycling	
Asleep	0.017	leisure, 5.5 mph	0.064
Badminton	0.097	leisure, 9.4 mph	0.100
Bakery, general (F)	0.035	racing	0.169
Basketball	0.138	Dancing	
Billards	0.042	ballroom	0.051
Bookbinding	0.038	choreographed,	
Boxing		twist, disco	0.168
in ring	0.222	Digging trenches	0.145
sparring	0.138	Dishwashing	0.033
Canoeing		Drawing (standing)	0.036
leisure	0.044	Eating (sitting)	0.023
racing	0.103	Electrical work	0.058
Card playing	0.025	Farming	
Carpentry, general	0.052	barn cleaning	0.135
Carpet sweeping (F)	0.045	driving harvester	0.040
Carpet sweeping (M)	0.048	driving tractor	0.037
Circuit-training	0.185	feeding animals	0.065
Cleaning (F)	0.062	feeding cattle	0.085
Cleaning (M)	0.058	forking straw bales	0.138
Climbing hills		milking by hand	0.054
with no load	0.121	milking by machine	0.023
with 5-kg load	0.129	shoveling grain	0.085
with 10-kg load	0.140	Field hockey	0.134
with 20-kg load	0.147	Fishing	0.062
Coal mining		Food shopping (F)	0.062
drilling coal, rock	0.094	Food shopping (M)	0.058
erecting supports	0.088	Football	0.132
shoveling coal	0.108	Forestry	
Cooking (F)	0.045	ax chopping, fast	0.297
Cooking (M)	0.048	ax chopping, slow	0.085
Cricket		barking trees	0.123
batting	0.083	carrying logs	0.186
bowling	0.090	felling trees	0.132
Croquet	0.059	hoeing	0.091

(Table continues on next page.)

TABLE 4 (*continued*)

ACTIVITY	KCAL / MIN KG	ACTIVITY	KCAL / MIN KG
planting by hand	0.109	cello (sitting)	0.041
sawing by hand	0.122	conducting	0.039
sawing, power	0.075	drums (sitting)	0.066
stacking firewood	0.088	flute (sitting)	0.035
trimming trees	0.129	horn (sitting)	0.029
weeding	0.072	organ (sitting)	0.053
Furriery	0.083	piano (sitting)	0.040
Gardening		trumpet (standing)	0.031
digging	0.126	violin (sitting)	0.045
hedging	0.077	woodwind (sitting)	0.032
mowing	0.112	Painting, inside	0.034
raking	0.054	Painting, outside	0.077
Golf	0.085	Planting seedlings	0.070
Gymnastics	0.066	Plastering	0.078
Horse-grooming	0.128	Printing	0.035
Horseback riding		Running, cross-country	0.163
galloping	0.137	Running, horizontal	
trotting	0.110	11 min, 30 sec per mile	0.135
walking	0.041	9 min per mile	0.193
Ironing (F)	0.033	8 min per mile	0.208
Ironing (M)	0.064	7 min per mile	0.228
Judo	0.195	6 min per mile	0.252
Knitting, sewing (F)	0.022	5 min 30 sec per mile	0.289
Knitting, sewing (M)	0.023	Scraping paint	0.063
Laundry	0.039	Scrubbing floors (F)	0.109
Locksmith	0.057	Scrubbing floors (M)	0.108
Lying still, awake	0.019	Shoe repair, general	0.045
Machine-tooling		Sitting quietly	0.021
machine	0.048	Skating	0.075
operating lathe	0.052	Skiing, hard snow	
operating punch press	0.088	level, moderate speed	0.119
tapping and drilling	0.065	level, walking	0.143
welding	0.052	uphill, maximum speed	0.274
working sheet metal	0.048	Skiing, soft snow	
Marching, rapid	0.142	leisure (F)	0.111
Mopping floor (F)	0.062	leisure (M)	0.098
Mopping floor (M)	0.058	Skindiving, as frogman	
Music playing		considerable motion	0.276
accordion (sitting)	0.032	moderate motion	0.206

TABLE 4 (*continued*)

ACTIVITY	KCAL / MIN KG	ACTIVITY	KCAL / MIN KG
Snowshoeing, soft snow	0.166	Table tennis	0.068
Squash	0.212	Tailoring	
Standing quietly (F)	0.025	cutting	0.041
Standing quietly (M)	0.027	hand-sewing	0.032
Steel mill, working in		machine-sewing	0.045
fettling	0.089	pressing	0.062
forging	0.100	Tennis	0.109
hand rolling	0.137	Typing	
merchant mill roll-	0.145	electric	0.027
removing slag	0.178	manual	0.031
tending furnace	0.126	Volleyball	0.050
tipping molds	0.092	Walking	
Stock clerking	0.054	3 mph	0.063
Swimming		4 mph	0.094
backstroke	0.169	Walking downstairs	0.048‡
breast stroke	0.162	Walking upstairs	0.144‡
crawl, fast	0.156	Wallpapering	0.048
crawl, slow	0.128	Watch repairing	0.025
side stroke	0.122	Window cleaning (F)	0.059
treading, fast	0.170	Window cleaning (M)	0.058
treading, normal	0.062	Writing (sitting)	0.029

Sources: Katch, F. I., & McArdle, W. D. *Nutrition, Weight Control and Exercise.* Boston: Houghton-Mifflin, 1977. Guthrie, H. A. *Introductory Nutrition.* St. Louis: Mosby, 1975. Variations from original table are author's extrapolations.
*As individuals become more obese they use relatively fewer calories per kg of body weight. If you are more than fifty pounds overweight, you may use only two-thirds of the energy estimated from this table. To get a more accurate estimate of your needs, deduct 5 percent of the total you obtain using this table for each ten pounds above desirable weight, up to a maximum of 30 percent for sixty pounds overweight and higher. An example using this table follows. To convert pounds to kg, divide by 2.2.
‡Comfortable pace.

During a period of weight maintenance, if a twenty-eight-day eating and activity record comes within 30 percent of matching, and the level of caloric intake is within 400 calories of the estimated calorie needs from table 3, you are not likely to deviate markedly from normal metabolism. But, if conscientious record keeping using the activity estimates is consistently more than 30 percent higher than an accurate eating record, and you are not losing weight, it

TABLE 5
Eating Record

	CALORIES	TOTALS
BREAKFAST		
2 slices whole wheat bread	140	
2 oz. cheese	200	
½ grapefruit (medium)	40	
coffee, 1 tsp. 2% milk	10	
Total	390	390
LUNCH		
large green salad, with ½ tomato, celery, carrot sticks, green pepper slices, and 1 can of tuna, water pack	250	
½ tbsp. Italian dressing	40	
2 slices whole wheat bread	140	
Total	430	820
SNACK		
medium apple	Total 60	880
DINNER		
6 oz. herbed pork, lean	400	
baked potato	90	
1 glass dry white wine	90	
4 dried figs	160	
orange	60	
1 oz. cheese	100	
Total	900	
	Grand total	1780

may be another indication of slow metabolism since these estimates assume normal requirements. Remember, of course, that both intake and expenditure estimates done in this way are very rough. The evidence is not strong unless you *consistently* find that your energy expenditure is 30 percent greater than your intake, averaged each week for a full four weeks, without weight loss.

During a weight loss period the difference between energy intake and energy expenditure should be approximately equal to the number of calories represented in your weight loss. After week

TABLE 6
Activity Record
Male, age 49*, wgt. 176 lbs. (80 kg), 20 lbs. overweight†

ACTIVITY AND TIME	NO. MINUTES × WGT. (KG) × calories per minute	APPROXIMATE CALORIES EXPENDED
8 hrs. sleeping	480 × 80 × .017	653
8 hrs. office work		
(4 hrs. writing,	240 × 80 × .029	557
4 hrs. sitting)	240 × 80 × .021	403
2 hrs. at meals	120 × 80 × .023	221
90 minutes stand-		
ing	90 × 80 × .027	194
30 minutes clean-		
ing up after		
dinner (equal		
to dishwash-		
ing)‡	30 × 80 × .033	79
45 minutes bath-		
room, washing,		
cleaning teeth,		
shower (equal		
to dishwash-		
ing)	45 × 80 × .033	119
1 hr. walking at 3		
mph (estab-		
lished from		
daily pedome-		
ter record, 3		
miles of a 6-		
mile total)	60 × 80 × .063	302
45 minutes walk-		
ing at 4 mph (3		
miles)	45 × 80 × .094	338
1 hr. sitting read-		
ing	50 × 80 × .021	101
30 min. lying in		
bed reading	30 × 80 × .019	46
		3013
		−603*†
	Estimated total expenditure	2410

*Deduct 10 percent for age-related decrease in metabolism for sedentary persons.
†Deduct 10 percent for degree of overweight.
‡If an activity is not represented in Table 4, use the estimates for an activity that is a near equivalent.

three of a diet, for every 3500 calories that your energy expenditure exceeds your caloric intake, you should lose a pound. Again, because of the inherent error in using "average" caloric expenditures and "average" caloric content from standard food and activity charts, a difference as large as 30 percent is possible. Part of this difference may in reality be due to some slight metabolic slowdown, and part due to your having relatively large fat mass. However, if you have been conscientious in your record keeping, a large (over 30 percent) deviation from expected weight loss over several weeks suggest a slower than average metabolism.

On the following pages I illustrate how an activity and eating diary are kept (tables 5 and 6). In your own notebook you can use the lefthand page for the eating record and the righthand page for your activity record. For self-evaluation purposes, it is not necessary to be more exact with respect to time spent in most of your activities if you lead a sedentary life. Three activities—sleeping, your occupation, and extra physical activity (walking, sports)—will account for about 80 percent of your caloric expenditure. In my example, note how important walking is. In just one hour and forty-five minutes, the time spent moving about in this man's day, he accounted for over 20 percent of his entire caloric needs in a twenty-four-hour period.

13

STAY FIT WITH VARIETY

Forty five minutes of walking and the Good Morning Routine provide a solid basis for fitness and weight management. Once you have your weight under control and feel what it's like to have the strength and energy to be fit, you may become interested in experimenting with a number of different physical activities and adding some variety to your daily routine. You have a lot to look forward to, and this is a chapter to help you get started.

Jogging

Ask confirmed joggers why they run thirty or more miles a week and they will tell you, plain and simple, that it is one of the most important things in their lives. They call it, using Dr. William Glasser's words, "A Positive Addiction." It makes them feel stronger, physically and mentally. It has a significance for them that only other joggers may be able to appreciate. They speak about it with a reverence comparable to that of devoutly religious individuals for whom prayer and meditation make life more meaningful.

I know what the addicted jogger is speaking about. While I enjoy tennis and bicycling, nothing compares with the satisfaction of a long run over mountain trails or an ocean beach. I have also discovered that nothing is so refreshing as a late afternoon jog around one of the beautiful Nashville parks. Contrary to what you might believe, it's when you have finished a grueling day at your desk, when you feel especially sluggish, that some sort of physical activity is most invigorating. Try scheduling your walks at that time, and if you experiment with jogging, see if a late afternoon run doesn't send you home feeling relaxed and refreshed instead of washed out and grouchy.

Notwithstanding my own preference for jogging over all other physical activities, I do not recommend it for overweight people at the start of a weight reduction program. The impact of each step brings three-to-four times your body weight crushing down on your lower extremities. When you add that impact pressure to slight deviations from good foot alignment or from good posture, both of which seem to be more prevalent among overweight individuals, you increase the chances of injury tremendously. If you start jogging before you are ready, your knees, ankles, feet, hips, or lower back may be damaged to such an extent that you will never be able to enjoy it.

In spite of the above warning, I include this section on jogging because it can ultimately become a source of great pleasure for formerly overweight people. Formerly fat people, especially those who were once extremely overweight and never athletic, probably experience more amazement and personal satisfaction from developing their potential to jog for forty-five minutes, or more, than any naturally thin person can ever appreciate. I also know that as a person approaches ideal weight, the urge to try to jog will hit almost everyone who has gotten fit enough to walk briskly for forty-five minutes. One day, someone will glide past you as you are out walking, and something about the way that person moves will stimulate you. Your feet will be pulled as though by some magnetic force and you will be hard put to restrain yourself.

Many excellent books on jogging have appeared in the last few years. I list a few in the bibliography that will add to what I have to say and answer specific questions about the physical aspects of running. However, these books do not attend to the special problems formerly overweight (possibly still even a little bit overweight) sedentary individuals face. And frequently, the main purpose of these books is to show readers how to develop their full running and fitness potential. Their focus is on how to get faster or train for a marathon. I have a different emphasis. I want to show you how to enjoy it. To do this, you must be able to make a transition from walking to jogging, stay injury free, and experience some mental transformation.

Before I describe my four-phase program for making this transition, I want to make a few observations about forty-five minutes of walking, as compared with forty-five minutes of jogging.

Forty-five minutes of walking is essential to your health and weight management. Without adding forty-five minutes of walking, an otherwise sedentary person will never be able to eat like a normal human being. Forty-five minutes of walking will improve your cardiovascular condition and add to your mental as well as physical energy and well-being.

Forty-five minutes of jogging is utterly unnecessary. Its only real physical advantage over walking is that it burns considerably more calories per unit time spent doing it. There is nothing to indicate that joggers are healthier than walkers. Sure, they build the capacity to move faster, but it's at a greatly increased risk of injury to their muscles, joints, and ligaments. Although they can move faster, this does not guarantee longer lives, or even greater protection from cardiac disease—only greater endurance for jogging. Furthermore, a person does not even need to jog forty-five minutes a day to achieve a high level of speed or cardiovascular endurance. Three times a week for about thirty minutes each time will do it. So, why forty-five minutes of jogging, and why almost every day?

People jog for forty-five minutes because it's an ego trip—one you can take almost every day, provided you don't overdo it. Being able to take an ego trip can play a very important role in your life, so I am not using these words disparagingly. In some mysterious way, being able to jog forty-five minutes or so with very little effort (something you *can* learn to do) and doing it five or more times a week seems to give people a sense of strength and self-confidence blended with tranquility and peace of mind that is rarely obtained from other activities. Those three periods per week of thirty minutes each that yield all anyone needs for physical fitness do not seem to produce the psychological benefits and rarely an addiction to physical activity. Most people who exercise only three times a week take it like a dose of medicine. Five or more days a week for at least forty-five minutes seems to be required for it to "get into your blood." And this, literally, may be exactly what happens. Jogging for such periods does produce a number of hormone changes, including changes in endorphins (a morphinelike substance) and catecholamines, both of which influence mental states. Whatever the reason, the net effect was put quite neatly by the runner who said, "People run because they like themselves better for doing it." Maybe you will, too.

The Foundation

My technique for learning to jog injury free and with pleasure will work for almost anyone without a physical handicap that makes jogging impossible. However, I strongly advise against making the easy transition from walking to jogging that I describe if you are more than 20 percent overweight. Get down below that figure first. Better yet, just keep building your walking program and try out some other activities, such as swimming or bicycling, until you get within 10 percent of your ideal weight. These activities are much less likely to cause weight-related injury to your muscles and joints.

You have to walk before you can run. Reach a comfortable forty-five minutes of walking, a good portion of it at a brisk four miles per hour pace. Once you have accomplished that time and pace, make it a part of your life for at least two full weeks. Doing it once without significant aches or pains is not enough. Give your body time to develop its strength and endurance before you start my four-phase jogging program.

THE FOUR-PHASE JOGGING PROGRAM

Phase I

1. Walk at your usual pace for about fifteen minutes.
2. Speed up to a brisk walk and hold for it for one or two minutes.
3. Break into an easy shuffle step or trot, *and actually slow down a bit from your fast walk.*
4. Shuffle along for one or two minutes at this somewhat slower pace than your brisk walk.
5. Slow to your three-miles-per-hour walking pace for one to two minutes.
6. Alternate shuffles with comfortable walking for about fifteen minutes.
7. Walk anyway you like for the last fifteen minutes.

In order to make an injury-free transition from walking to jogging, and in order for you to discover that reserve power for the long distance you can ultimately reach, you actually go slower with your first jogging steps than you can move in a brisk walk. If you do not violate this important principle in your first few weeks of jogging, chances are you will never number yourself among that 60 percent of runners who report running-related injuries.

But why, at first, go slower than you can go walking? Because the jogging motion requires more effort, and it is quite different from walking in many mechanical aspects. You will feel it differently over your entire body, especially in the legs and lower back. You will also find yourself holding your arms and upper body differently, possibly tighter, so stay relaxed.

You will probably be using more energy in the slow jog than in your brisk walk. You will know by your breathing rate, or your pulse rate if you measure it. Keep your effort as close to that of brisk walking as possible. Do not get yourself completely out of breath (or as high as 90 percent of your maximum heart rate, see table 1 in chapter six). Speed is absolutely not important at this stage.

Experiment with your stride. Each person will have a length that suits his or her physical equipment. Usually, rather short steps feel best and are more efficient. Short steps keep your center of gravity well over your foot placement and you do not have to strain to push or pull your body along. However, some people do feel better with a rather long stride. That's why you experiment.

Don't try to run on your toes—that's for sprinters. Land naturally, heel first, or almost flat footed. As long as you don't push yourself, your body is likely to choose the technique that really is best for it. Jogging is as natural a movement as walking. For many people, it may actually feel better.

TARGET FOR PHASE I

For the middle fifteen of your forty-five minutes of activity, alternate minutes of trotting with walking for as many days as it takes to get comfortable and to determine that your muscles and joints are not going to react negatively. No matter how good it feels, do not go to Phase II for at least two weeks. Remember that this may be the first time since childhood that you have ever done five or ten minutes of running in a fifteen-minute period. Just because you can do it once doesn't mean your body has become conditioned well enough to go longer or faster. Let your muscles build and your bones and joints get stronger. Be patient.

Phase II

1. Walk for ten minutes.

2. Gradually increase your walk/jog time from fifteen minutes to thirty minutes. But, hold each jog period to no more than two minutes. Take about two weeks to reach a total of thirty minutes.

3. Walk five minutes to cool down.

4. About now you will know whether jogging tends to make you stiffer, either right afterwards or the next day. If it does, five minutes of stretching (numbers one through eight of the Good Morning Routine) will help. More and more runners are discovering that stretching after a run is the most important time for this activity. And each morning, do not neglect the Good Morning Routine. It, too, will protect you.

TARGET FOR PHASE II

Your goal is to reach a full thirty minutes alternating walking with jogging. I know you will want to go faster and to go longer than two minutes in each jogging cycle. Great. You are motivated. But, don't. You may have the cardiovascular capacity for more speed or distance, but if this is the first major physical activity in your life, it's your bones, joints, and muscles that are not ready. Going faster and longer too soon is an almost certain route to aches and pains, especially if you are still ten or twenty pounds overweight. Once you reach thirty minutes, stay with it for another two weeks before going to Phase III.

Instead of stiffness, you may find yourself feeling a few aches and pains with this amount of walking and jogging each day. This may be a sign that you aren't stretching enough after your jog, or, that alternating days with different activities will be best for you. Try using the walk/jog routine only three days a week and walk or play active games on the others.

Remember, jogging is not essential to your health. If you hurt, swimming, bicycling, or active games may be more suitable to your physical equipment.

Phase III

1. Warm up with five minutes of walking.

2. During your thirty minute walk/jog periods, gradually increase your jogging time from two, to three, to four minutes, and on upwards. However, when you walk, hold those periods to no more than two minutes.

3. Save at least five minutes for walking to cool down and another five minutes for stretching. Stiffness, aches, or pains can be helped by more stretching after your jog and each morning after you get up.

TARGET FOR PHASE III

Your goal is to reach a full thirty minutes of gentle nonstop jogging. It doesn't matter how many days or weeks it takes for you to reach this goal, and, for that matter, you need never do it for your health. Just keep on walking, and if you like, jog occasionally, as long as it feels good.

Definitely adopt alternate walking and jogging days if you experience significant muscle soreness or joint pain. You will reach thirty minutes of continuous jogging just about as soon doing it on alternate days as you will doing it every day. You *can* take a day off, and running may prove to be more pleasurable if you sprinkle in a little tennis, swimming, or other activities. Alternating activities permits the muscles involved in jogging to fully recover, which may take as long as forty-eight hours for some people.

Once you reach thirty minutes of continuous jogging, three or more days a week, stay with it for at least two more weeks before going on to Phase IV.

Phase IV

You have finally reached the point when you can crack the barriers that stand in the way of discovering whether you will experience the joy of running that its enthusiasts rave about.

It is extremely important that you do not jump into Phase IV too quickly. If you cannot do about thirty minutes of gentle jogging, and if you have not been doing it regularly for at least two weeks, you do not have either the physical or mental preparation for the last step. Not only is it dangerous to overtax yourself, but you will be disappointed.

Up to now, you may occasionally have had the urge to go faster. At other times, in contrast, you may have felt just the opposite—that you had to discipline yourself to get out and walk or jog. But everything up to now has only been preparation for the present phase. When you do the two things I now suggest you will discover whether jogging will have the same meaning to you that it has for those who call it a positive addiction.

There are two steps in Phase IV.

1. *One day each week,* after you have warmed up, about twenty minutes into your jog, *go faster.* Run a couple of hundred yards as fast as you feel like (but *not* top speed). Go back to your gentle jog (not a walk) until you get your breath back. This will illustrate that you can actually recover while still jogging. Repeat your faster run at least four times. Work hard—see just how strong you are—actually get out of breath. After you've finished these four sprints, cool down slowly by jogging for about five minutes.

2. On other running days, gradually increase your time until you reach approximately forty-five minutes. On these days, stay slow, but feel free to play around. Look for different surfaces to run on, some trails, a track, some hills. One other day each week, see how it feels to build to as much as an hour of jogging, but be sure to keep it comfortable.

Do not do a high intensity period of running more than once a week if you want to avoid injury.

TARGET FOR PHASE IV

Your goal is to build the reserve that makes forty-five minutes of jogging feel like child's play, and then to maintain that capacity all of your life.

By going faster, near 90 percent of your capacity, once a week, you make your gentle jog something that can be done at only 60–70 percent of your cardiovascular capacity. Right now, as a sedentary overweight person, you will have to use your imagination to appreciate the contrast: right now you may be using more than 70 percent of your capacity to walk at three miles per hour. In fact, it is quite likely that walking briskly—four miles per hour—would soon exhaust you. This four-phase jogging program makes jogging easier in terms of the cardiovascular effort required than walking is for you at the present time. You won't even be breathing hard. In other words, it will feel unbelievably easy because your heart will be beating more slowly jogging than it now does when you walk.

By increasing your jogging to a full hour at a gentle pace, just once a week, you make going for only forty to forty-five minutes on the other days seem very short. The psychological effect lies in the feeling you have of wanting more. You begin to plan for that one day each week when you have the time for a special run. On the physical side, one longer day builds the endurance capacity of your legs which makes the physical work of forty-five minutes of jogging seem lighter.

Summary

In the early weeks, building the capacity for effortless, pleasurable jogging requires a great deal of self-discipline. At first, it isn't effortless, and it may not be particularly pleasurable because it still feels like hard work. It's your anticipation of things to come as you get better and jogging gets easier that keeps you going. You may also discover how jogging increases your control over your weight by burning more calories than walking. While that is often by itself not enough to keep people jogging, it adds to one's other motivations.

When you persevere through the first three phases, you build the foundation for both speed and endurance. When you add a little more speed on one day, and a little more time on another in Phase IV, you build a reserve cushion that makes ordinary effort feel easy. This is the basis for the psychological experiences that make running so pleasant for the committed jogger.

As you begin to vary your runs, you will find that your mind responds differently to different levels of intensity and that, depending on what you want to experience as you jog, or after, you have a great deal of control. Some days you may want to work out a problem as you jog—you loaf along so you can concentrate.

Other times, you get the urge to test yourself by going faster or up hills—that's exhilarating. Sometimes you just start moving and let things happen—the mind roves with the body, and that's refreshing.

Running is a personal experience. Its mental and emotional effects can not be communicated very precisely from one person to another. Those of us who enjoy it—well, we can only say it feels good and we feel somehow better for doing it. It's only when you have progressed through the first three phases of training to the level of Phase IV that you are physically and mentally equipped to discover whether jogging is going to have any special meaning for you. It's unfortunate, perhaps, but it's impossible to find this out unless you are willing to go through that probationary period—and it may take six months to a year.

ALTERNATE EXERCISES

Strength Training

Here is a special set of dumbbell exercises (you can use books) that you can add to or alternate with the ones in the Good Morning Routine.

Dumbbell Rowing (for the upper back)   With a dumbbell in each hand, knees slightly bent, bend forward until your upper body is parallel to the floor. Hold the dumbbells at arm's length directly below the shoulder, palms facing rear. Raise dumbbells by driving the elbow up and to the rear (avoid using your biceps—let the elbows lead).

You can raise both arms together, or alternate. You can turn palms to face your body for variety. Breathe normally and repeat at a comfortable moderate pace until you feel the strain (about ten or twelve times).

Standing Press (for the shoulders and back of arms)   With dumbbells at shoulder length, palms forward, push up over head to full extension. Lower. Move at a slow to moderate pace. Some days, do both arms up and down simultaneously, other days, alternate. About ten to twelve times.

Flys (for chest and shoulders)   Lie flat on floor (knees can be

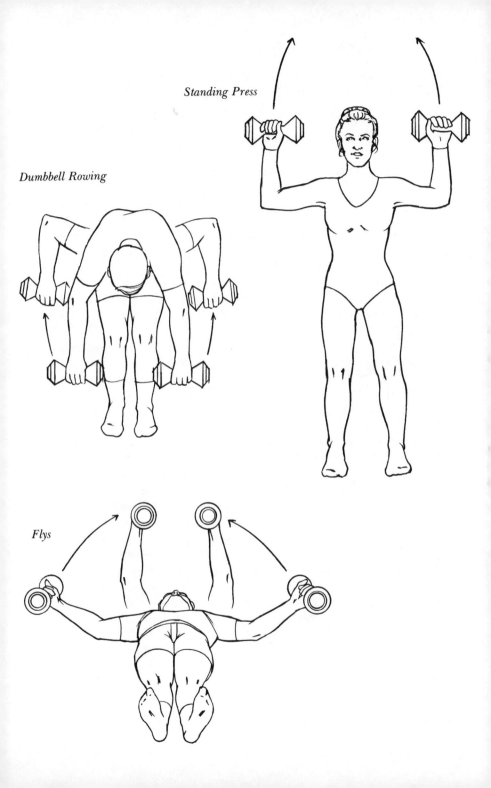

Standing Press

Dumbbell Rowing

Flys

straight or bent), dumbbell in each hand, arms outstretched to sides, palms up. The movement is like a flying motion: with arms slightly bent at elbows, raise the bells to top position directly above the chest, return to floor position. Start with only as many as you can handle until you feel the strain. Add one per week until you can do at least ten. This exercise and the next are two of the better ones for the chest muscles. If you use a light weight, be sure to do enough to feel it.

Overhead Flys (chest, shoulders, and arms)   Lie flat, arms next to sides, dumbbells in palms facing in. With elbows very slightly bent, slowly raise arms, up and back over your head toward the floor. You do not have to touch the floor behind you with the bells. Return to starting position. Inhale as you raise; exhale as you return to position. This is a rather strenuous exercise and taxes much of the upper body. You may do only one or two to begin with. It can be done standing, in which case it uses the shoulder muscles a little more than the pectorals and feels somewhat easier.

Floor Press (shoulders and chest)   Flat on back, elbows out to side at shoulder height. Upper arm is flat on floor, forearm bent at ninety degrees, palms face forward. Press up (arms completely extended at shoulder height). Then return upper arms to floor (forearm remains bent at ninety degrees). Repeat ten to twelve times, or until you feel the strain.

Improvisation   Lifting light weights has a very stimulating effect on your system. If you use them in continuous motion as you walk around your house, making whatever movement strikes your fancy, you get an effect that cannot be duplicated by any other form of exercise. Five minutes' worth will leave you breathing faster and tingling all over. Keep the intensity of this following workout moderate. It's a good one for alternate days.

Be inventive. As you walk, press bells up from the shoulders, make slow punching motions forward, then forward and up. Stop and do the shoulder threesome. Start walking and do bicep curls. Hold your arms out to the front or sides, and rotate your palms. In five minutes you will have had quite a workout. This is a good workout to do in the morning if you still feel sleepy fifteen minutes after you've gotten up. Try it while you're waiting for the toast, or for your pot of coffee to perk.

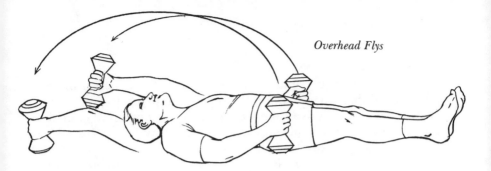

Overhead Flys

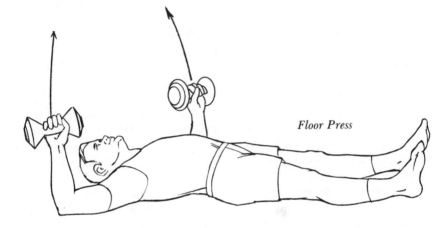

Floor Press

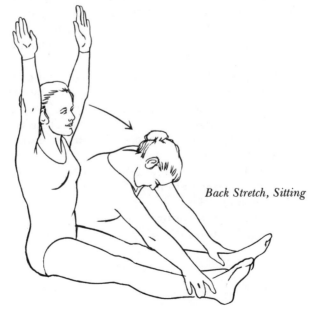

Back Stretch, Sitting

Yoga

In addition to obtaining marvelous flexibility benefits, many people find that yoga provides them with the psychological experience that others derive from long gentle jogs or a period of meditation. Yoga is a discipline that integrates mind and body. It's more than stretching—it can be a way of life.

The practice of yoga leads to self-control and greater body awareness. I describe here a few yogic-style exercises to add variety to your Good Morning Routine. I list some books in the bibliography that have helped many people develop a well-rounded yogic practice on their own. A full understanding of the spiritual and physical aspects of yoga requires a great deal of study and most people will profit from having a teacher.

Back Stretch, Sitting People with lower back problems generally must avoid bending forward at the waist in the standing position with straight legs. The standing back stretch requires lifting the upper body against the force of gravity, which can aggravate back problems. You avoid danger in the sitting position and have greater control over the stretch.

Sit on the floor, legs together stretched in front. Raise your arms up over your head as you take a deep breath. Gently bend forward from the hips. Exhale as you reach for your legs as far forward as possible without straining. Holding on to your knees, calves, ankles, or feet (whatever is comfortable keeping your legs straight), let your body relax into the stretch. Keep breathing normally in this position and hold for a count of twenty.

You have several options in this stretch. You can hold it once for as much as a minute or more, relaxing into the stretching position, not straining. Or, you can take a deep breath, lifting your arms up over your head as you return to the upright position, and then repeat the forward bend as above. It can be done several times, slowly, about twenty seconds each stretch.

When you reach the upright position with arms over your head, you can lean back several inches for a few seconds to strengthen your abdominal muscles.

With practice, you will find yourself able to reach farther and farther forward, but don't rush to reach your toes. Stretch, don't strain.

Sitting Twist Another excellent exercise for the lower back done gently. As with all yogic stretches, it takes many months to develop enough flexibility to perform the exercise in its extreme position and the student must have patience to advance at a pace appropriate to his or her own capability. The following description is for the first, or elementary position of the twist.

On the floor, in the sitting position, begin with both legs together, extended. Bend the right leg at the knee, placing the right foot to the outside of the left knee.

Turn to the right, placing your right hand directly behind you, fairly close to your body.

Place your left elbow to the outside of your right knee, exerting just a little pressure and turn your head to look behind you. Line your chin up with your right shoulder.

You may feel the stretch in any or all of a number of places, depending upon where your ligaments or muscles are stiffest—hips, lower back, thigh, or shoulder. Relax into the stretch holding for a count of twenty, which gives enough time for the tightest areas to loosen and lengthen. Do not bounce, push, or thrust in any yogic-style stretch. Keep breathing naturally.

Reverse legs and twist to the other side.

One long stretch is enough. But, as with the sitting stretch above, many people gain added benefit from up to three slow repetitions. Each feels better than the last and you can see your flexibility increase more dramatically.

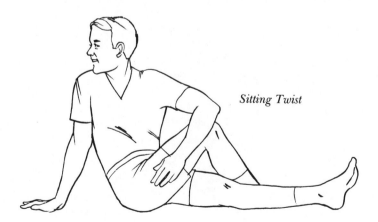

Sitting Twist

Knee and Thigh Stretch On floor in sitting position, bring the soles of your feet together close to your body, knees out to the side. Grasp feet firmly with your hands, and, sitting as erect as possible, pull your feet a little closer to the body. Slowly lower your knees as far as is comfortable towards the floor, continuing to clasp your feet. Hold position for a count of twenty. Then, relax the effort to push your knees to the floor for a few moments, maintaining the position in other respects. Then, try to reach the floor again with your knees (another count of twenty).

Relax. Extend your legs forward. You may want to flex them a few times and rotate your feet at the ankles.

Half Back Pushup Lie on your back, arms at side. Raise yo pelvis high in the air by bringing your feet back up, flat on th floor, close to your body. (Your lower legs will form a ninety degree

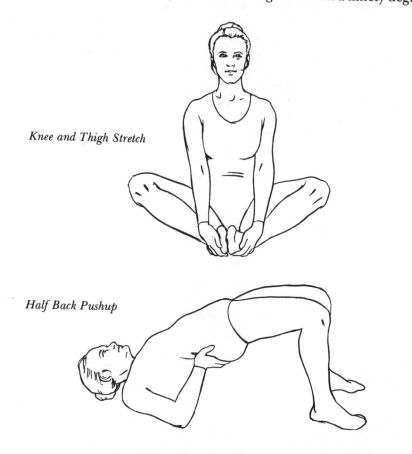

Knee and Thigh Stretch

Half Back Pushup

angle to the floor.) Place your hands under your hips for support. Keep your shoulders, neck, and head on the floor. Hold it for twenty seconds without forcing the extension.

While this exercise helps maintain spinal flexibility, it should not be done by people with chronic back pain without physician's permission.

Cobra   Lie on your stomach, face to one side, arms at side. Bring your hands next to your shoulders, place them flat on the floor, fingers facing forward. Turn your head to the front, lift your forehead, letting your chin just touch the floor.

Then, without help from your arms, raise your head, shoulders, and chest as far as possible, trying to look back over your head. When you reach the limit, add some help from your arms. You are trying to flex your spine, so be sure to leave your pelvis flat on the floor. Curve only the upper body from the waist up as far as it will go without undue strain. Hold for several seconds breathing natural.

Return to the prone position, head to the side, arms at sides, and relax. Breathe normally.

Repeat up to three times.

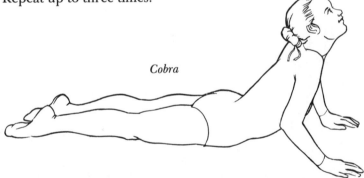

Cobra

Shoulder Stand   This is a superb exercise for the circulation. It can aid in the relief of aches and edema in the legs. According to yogic teachings, it can stimulate the thyroid gland and aid in the control of obesity. (Unfortunately, I know of no research to confirm this claim.)

The main purpose of this exercise is to elevate the legs to a position higher than the heart. If you have high blood pressure, you must check with your physician the extent to which you can perform the shoulder stand. Most likely he will okay a simple elevation and not a full shoulder stand. In such cases, lying flat on your back, you can place your feet and lower legs on a footstool or chair and relax. Another position suitable for those people who cannot do a full shoulder stand is to wiggle up to a wall, getting your rear end as close to it as possible, and extending your legs upward using the wall for support.

To accomplish a full shoulder stand, lie flat on your back, arms at side. Bring your knees up to your chest and roll slightly backwards to raise your rear from the floor. Place your hands firmly behind your hips (as high on the sides of your lower back as possible) for support.

Begin to straighten your legs. The ultimate goal is to reach a position with the legs pointing towards the ceiling. However, many people find that they cannot extend that far vertically. In such cases, it's perfectly okay to keep a slight bend in the back or, for that matter, to keep your knees bent and your body in a curled position. You are still getting plenty of benefit. You will feel the relief in your legs.

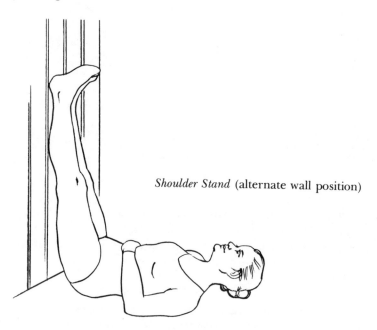

Shoulder Stand (alternate wall position)

In the fully extended position you support yourself with your hands; your upper arms, shoulders, neck, and head are flat against the floor.

You can hold this position for a full minute or more. You can do creative things by moving your legs—side to side, back and forth. You can bend your knees to resume a curled position and then return to the extended position. When you add variation in this way you can hold the position for several minutes and increase its benefits.

Yogic Relaxation Position   When you add the positions I have just described to the stretches (not the weight work) in the Good Morning set, you have a full beginner's yoga routine that can take twenty to thirty minutes.

Done at an unhurried pace, focusing your mind on your body sensations, twenty to thirty minutes of yoga yield physical and mental relaxation that cannot be excelled by any other method.

The perfect way to end a session is with the relaxation pose. Once you have practiced the pose and the focusing that goes with it, you can use the position for relaxation purposes at any time. Yoga teachers claim that just a few minutes in this position can be as refreshing as several hours of sleep. Whether or not this is true, I cannot say, but I can verify that even two minutes will make you feel calm and refreshed.

Lie flat on your back. If you like, your head can be elevated about an inch on a folded towel or book. Your legs should be fully extended, feet separated about six inches. Let your arms lie flat, a bit to the side, palms up.

Take a couple of full deep breaths, exhale completely on each. Resume normal breathing.

Focus your attention on your toes. Just think, "Let loose, relax." Linger there several seconds. Let your awareness settle on your soles and arches—think, "Relax." Wander up to your ankles. You need only to think, "Calm," and concentrate for a few seconds on each body part. Proceed to your calves, knees, thighs—slowly, no rush. Breathe naturally. Focus on your pelvis, hips, stomach, chest— slowly, one at a time. You are sending your body the order, "Let loose." Travel next to your fingers and work up to your hands, lower arms, upper arms, shoulder, and neck. Release the tension. If the urge to wiggle something strikes you, do it. It aids the process of letting go. Then, concentrate on letting loose throughout your face: your forehead, eyes, cheeks, lips, teeth, tongue. Your lips can be slightly parted.

The *doing* of relaxation lies in the attitude of *not doing;* it is, in fact, an *undoing*—letting yourself become aware of your body and letting go of yourself. If your mind wanders as you focus on your

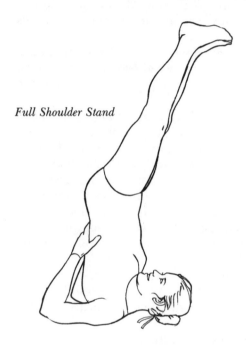

Full Shoulder Stand

Yogic Relaxation Position

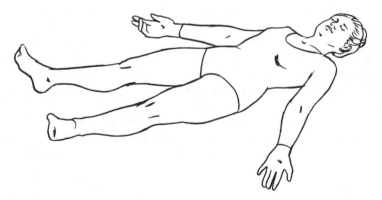

body, just bring it back gently, like a good shepherd dog guides the stray lamb back to the flock.

One of my yoga instructors always finished the session with a form of relaxation similar to what I have described, with suitable music playing softly in the background. If you try the relaxation pose with music, you may be very reluctant to rouse yourself when you finish.

Getting the Most out of an Exercise Facility

I must admit to a bias when it comes to choosing a health club or exercise facility. I have visited a number and have been given a few of the hard sells that certain spas are noted for. I have been impressed by some very expensive equipment and some very expensive clubs. But my preference remains for the YMCA. That is where I recommend you look first for facilities, classes, personal evaluation, and individual exercise supervision.

However, YMCA facilities vary, and some spas offer first-rate programs. Here's what to look for.

1. *Professional leadership.* Be sure the person in charge of the fitness program is fully trained in physical education. Many of your expensive spas, as well as your bargain basement clubs, use poorly trained part-time help as leaders. They will have little idea how to help an overweight and out-of-condition person get the most out of a class or a conditioning program. They know a single routine done at a single pace (the one that suits them best, not the participants). Sometimes, if they are not trying to get through their routine as quickly as possible, they use the time to show off, or for their own conditioning purposes. You can spot this attitude the first time you see it, but it may not be exhibited until you have bought your membership.

2. *Professional evaluation.* You can depend upon the validity of a YMCA physical fitness evaluation. The person in charge will have been professionally trained, or, if he or she is still in training, the supervisor will be near by. The Y has no ax to grind—they don't need to make you look good or bad to sell you a program. This may not be true of many commercial operations. I recall a visit to one of the most expensive spas in Nashville. My guide, who did not

know my profession, made a quick caliper measurement of my triceps skin fold, glanced at his chart, and said I had 25 percent body fat (that's more than double the true figure). For a moment I said nothing as he went on to describe the evaluation I would get if I joined. At one point he fingered his chart and noted that fifty sit-ups per minute would qualify me as "average." (He boasted that he did over one hundred.) This particular spa evidently uses the "make you look bad" strategy to convince you of how much you need their program. The "norms" on their charts were simply fictions, and this man knew nothing about measuring body fat. I told him so.

3. *Available facilities.* Many clubs sell far more memberships than their facilities can comfortably handle. Much of the time, this may work out okay for both the club and the avid exerciser since the majority of club members will rarely use the facilities. Before you join, visit the facility on several occasions at the times you will most likely use it. If you find patrons lined up waiting for a turn at the equipment, no place to sit in the sauna, and the indoor track (if they have one) looking like a subway platform at Times Square during rush hour, you may want to reconsider.

4. *Appropriate classes and instruction.* There are many enjoyable ways to get fit, and top flight facilities will offer, in addition to the usual fitness classes, a variety of different style dance classes, yoga, and games. More and more people are enrolling in aerobic dance, dancercise, or jazzercise, ballet, clogging, and square dancing, and getting a workout that can make an experienced runner breathless. You are likely to find a variety of such classes offered at the Y and, in some cities, at community centers under the Department of Parks and Recreation.

It can be valuable to know whether the leader has experience with overweight individuals and leads the class in such a way that no matter what your level of skill or fitness, you will be able to go at your own pace and benefit from your participation. If you can, observe the class before you join, or talk to someone who has been in it. After you have followed the program I suggest for twelve weeks, you are very likely to have more strength, flexibility, and cardiovascular endurance than the average beginner, as well as many advanced members of such classes. You will have a good foundation on which to add the specific dance skills.

Dancing is fun. It can become the focus of a fitness program. It can also be an excellent alternate activity in a program that features variety.

Be Your Own Person

If you are like most overweight and formerly inactive people, you are probably expecting to feel ill-coordinated and uncomfortable in any kind of activity group. Chances are you will feel much less this way if you get on the ball, lose twenty to thirty pounds in the next few months, and practice my all-around conditioning program during this time. You will be amazed at how your condition will compare with others in the group.

You may still feel that you have a poor sense of timing, and you may find yourself comparing your abilities with others in the group. It is certainly much easier for me to say "Stop comparing" than it is for you to switch your feelings on and off at command. Nevertheless, your attitude about yourself and the group may determine how much you get out of it. Cultivate a non-critical approach, both toward yourself, and as much as possible, the others in the group including the leader. Approach any class or fitness group with an openness to learn and an acceptance of your own physical limitations. Consider it an experiment. When you move, focus on your bodily sensations, just as though you were at home, doing one of your own routines. Most people find much more enjoyment from any sort of activity class when they stop comparing themselves with others and start enjoying the feelings of the moment. Avoid any sort of competition until you are in competitive shape.

The Racquet Sports

Some people find racquet sports more satisfying than walking, jogging, swimming, bicycling, or dancing. They enjoy the companionship and they like the skill and strategy involved. For many years, tennis was my daily activity. Playing at what might be called advanced intermediate level, you can obtain cardiovascular benefits with racquet sports, and burn calories, at least equivalent to walking at a moderate pace.

But each activity requires its own skills and yields its own special benefit. Conditioning is, to a large extent, specific. That is, you can develop considerable endurance for one activity—for example, jogging—yet find yourself getting breathless swimming one length of the pool. If you play singles tennis daily and take the game seriously enough to learn it to a level where you can enter local tournaments, you will have built the cardiovascular endurance to jog a couple of miles—but it won't feel easy or particularly good. You must train for each activity, developing the specific physical capacity and special skills in order to get the most enjoyment out of it.

With racquet sports, you will progress faster with lessons. In order to get good enough to get physical fitness benefits, you have to play several times a week. If you don't become proficient, you will spend most of your time standing around or picking up balls, which expends only about half the energy of steady walking.

The most useful advice I can give the beginner in any competitive sport is to avoid being supercritical toward yourself. Just focus your entire concentration on the ball, where you want it to go. Let your body go about its work in whatever way comes natural, exerting as little conscious control as possible. You'll play your best "unconscious," but focused on the ball. And when you are trying to learn a new stroke—any new body movement for that matter—concentrate on only one thing at a time. If you try to do more, you will get tense and frustrated.

To cultivate the correct mental attitude, I suggest you read *The Inner Game of Tennis* by Timothy Gallwey. Using tennis as an example, he presents a full exposition of the philosophy and techniques for learning and enjoying any competitive sport. As you go about learning to hit the ball where you want it to go, you may also learn a philosophy and technique for a more enjoyable as well as effective life.

How About a Bicycle?

A bicycle trip on weekends can be a welcome break from your other activities. Even if your city streets are crowded on weekdays, Sunday traffic is frequently light enough to make a city tour safe and interesting. If a city tour does not appeal to you, you can head straight for the countryside and discover different features of your area impossible to find or appreciate by foot or car. I have the county road maps of Tennessee (as well as of several states I have visited)* and look forward to a Saturday or a Sunday trip over back

*You can purchase county road maps from your State Highway or Transportation Department.

roads not illustrated on state maps. It's a way to be alone, enjoy the scenery, and end up in a park or historic community far off the beaten track for a picnic lunch.

I added bicycling to my activities just three years ago. It has had an exciting effect on my vacations. I have peddled over the Continental Divide, in the western parks, and down part of the Atlantic coast. I stay overnight at a motel, or just use a campsite in a park as home base and tour the area. There is nothing quite like a long glide from the top of a mountain or a plateau to the valley below. And with a good ten- or twelve-speed bicycle equipped with a special low ratio climbing gear, you can peddle back up the mountains at a comfortable slow pace that doesn't require much more effort than walking. When you add some bicycling to your vacations, you will come home weighing less than when you left.

If you bicycle along the coast or across the plains, you may have the exciting experience of being carried for miles by a breeze just strong enough to move you at your desired speed. You may go several miles without moving a peddle, like a sail boat. Of course, heading into such a wind is another story.

A bicycle is a very efficient machine. In order to get exercise equivalent to walking, jogging, or swimming, you have to put in more time, and, as far as I'm concerned, frequently go faster than I care to go. If you become an expert rider, you can, of course, obtain a degree of cardiovascular conditioning equal to the best runners or cross-country skiers. But most people don't care to use a bicycle this way. For them, as for me, it's a day off. I don't think I burn many more calories in three hours of bicycling than I do in an hour's jog.

If you don't know how to ride, it's never too late to learn. One of the best ways is to approach your local bicycle club (you can find out if you have one in your community by calling a bicycle shop). If your club is anything like ours in Nashville, some of its members will be eager to help you learn. They may have spare bicycles for you to learn on. In this way, you can see if you like bicycling without making an investment. Your club will most likely sponsor guided trips around your area every Saturday and Sunday—short or long, easy or difficult—something for every ability and taste. On some of these trips you may break for breakfast or lunch along the way and enjoy some local specialty.

If you already know how to ride, but haven't for years, the technique will come back to you in a matter of minutes. Try a friend's bicycle, or go to a bicycle shop where you can try out several models. When you are ready to buy one, you will do best at a bicycle shop, not a department or hardware store. If the sales person is a biker (they usually are), they will help you select one to suit your use.

There are many excellent brands of bicycles, which, in my opinion, are fairly equivalent at matching prices up to around $300. I think you can find a suitable model for as low as $150. Above $300, each brand will begin to offer special features that usually matter only to experienced riders who have special purposes in mind.

Don't be afraid to make a reasonable investment—if you keep a $250–300 bicycle in good condition, you can plan on selling it, should you want to, for as much as 75 percent of your purchase price several years down the road.

As for indoor exercise (stationary) bicycles, odds are you will rarely use one if you buy it—even if you set it up in front of the TV. Most people find them dreadfully boring. However, if you decide to try one, don't buy the cheap discount house variety. They don't hold up and they are hard to adjust to the amount of effort you desire. I can vouch for three good brands of stationary cycles— Tunturi, Monarch, and Schwinn. The booklet that comes with them will tell you how to ride for fitness benefits. If you do not set the resistance high enough, or peddle fast enough, to get your heart rate up as high as it would in a brisk walk or jog, you aren't getting a great deal of benefit from indoor cycling.

Swimming

Many physical education specialists rate swimming as the best all-around exercise. With the support provided by the water, there is little likelihood of joint injury and the swimming motion provides exercise for more muscle groups than do jogging, walking, or bicycling. In order to get significant cardiovascular benefits, and to burn as many calories as you do in forty-five minutes of brisk walking, you have to learn to swim well enough to keep at it continuously for almost the same amount of time. That is, for most people, swimming at a comfortable pace burns only a few more calories than brisk walking.

Most people cannot swim continuously for very long. It takes practice to reach the point where you can expend energy in swimming to equal that of a brisk walk. Thus, you have to work at it and if you think you would like swimming but don't do it very well, lessons will be helpful. Investigate your YMCA or a local swimming club. At these facilities you will also find classes in "water yoga" or more vigorous "watercise," both of which may do you much good if you're prone to joint pain or injury. If you combine some water exercises with more leisurely swimming, you will get a good workout in forty-five minutes.

Many overweight people come to enjoy swimming more than any other activity because their body fat (at least until they lose their extra stores) makes staying afloat easier than it is for thin people. For the overweight person, swimming, in just a matter of a few days, can become as effortless as a gentle jog for a thin person after weeks or months of practice. One of my patients who became an excellent swimmer combines three sessions a week with alternate days walking. She speaks of her swimming with the same mystical overtones as the addicted long distance runner speaks of running. Often, relaxed by the easy rhythm of her motions as she glides through the water, she enters a trancelike state, becomes oblivious to time, and completely absorbed in her body. She feels as though she is floating through clouds in space. When she first told me about her experience, her eyes misted over and the feelings sounded so good I wished I could get to be as expert a swimmer as she is. But I knew she had been hooked, just as I am with jogging. I knew that staying in shape was going to be a lot easier with feelings like those to look forward to, rather than another day of dieting.

EPILOGUE

Some people call me on the telephone to inquire about treatment and ask, "What is your success rate?" I answer, "One hundred percent for those who do what I say and zero for those who don't." Even more often, people make an appointment and after giving me their impression of where the problem lies, say, "I've tried everything and your program is my last hope. Can you help me?" I say, "No—I'd really, really like to, but I can't."

I say these things to make a point in the most dramatic way I know how. I don't have enough control over anyone's life to *make* them do what it takes to get slim and fit. I think I'd be afraid of that kind of power, even if it were available. After I've made one of those statements, I go on to tell prospective patients the same things I tell you: if you want to change, but feel weak and powerless to do so, I can, as I've done in the preceding pages, show you what to do to get stronger. As I pointed out, it's very much like practicing a musical instrument to develop your skill, or lifting weights to build muscles. You must do certain tasks each day—each one in and of itself is not hard. But they must be done. By doing them day after day, the benefits add up until you get stronger. It's automatic. It's an unavoidable consequence, just as getting physically stronger is an automatic, unavoidable consequence of lifting weights. In this book, I have shown you what you need to do to develop what we commonly call willpower and how to change a way of life that keeps you fat.

So the question is put to you: Will you *do* the things it takes to "get stronger?" It means using consistently one or more behavior change strategies to control your eating while losing weight, and possibly thereafter, if you can really outeat a reasonable level of physical activity. But most of all, it means getting in that extra forty-five minutes a day of physical activity, burning up those two hundred extra calories that stand between your present way of life and permanent weight control.

Slimness and fitness are unavoidable consequences of the behaviors I tell you to practice on a daily basis. The choice is yours: You can keep on looking for a miracle diet and periodically starve yourself for the rest of your life, continuing to feel guilty about your eating habits, or you can learn to eat sensibly and get active. I hope you will choose the latter. If you do, there is a very good chance that six months, a year, maybe as long as two years from now, you will look back in disbelief. It will have become easier and much more fun to live the daily life of a thin person, doing the things that keep you thin and fit, than it ever was to be fat.

APPENDICES

BIBLIOGRAPHY

APPENDIX A

Suggested Body Weights

HEIGHT	RANGE OF ACCEPTABLE WEIGHT	
	MEN	WOMEN
(feet-inches)	(pounds)	(pounds)
4'10"		92–119
4'11"		94–122
5'0"		96–125
5'1"		99–128
5'2"	112–41	102–31
5'3"	115–44	105–34
5'4"	118–48	108–38
5'5"	121–52	111–42
5'6"	124–56	114–46
5'7"	128–61	118–50
5'8"	132–66	122–54
5'9"	136–70	126–58
5'10"	140–74	130–63
5'11"	144–79	134–68
6'0"	148–84	138–73
6'1"	152–89	
6'2"	156–94	
6'3"	160–99	
6'4"	164–204	

Source: HEW Conference on Obesity, 1973.
Note: Height without shoes; weight without clothes.

APPENDIX B*

Sources and Functions of Major Nutrients

BEST SOURCES	FUNCTIONS	DEFICIENCY SYMPTOMS	RISKS OF OVERCONSUMPTION
	PROTEIN		
Fish, meat, poultry, eggs, cheese, and milk provide large amounts of easily utilized protein. The protein in legumes, nuts, seeds, and whole grains is incomplete. These foods should be eaten in combinations, one with another, or with a small amount of a complete protein food (meat, milk, or cheese) to enhance their biological value.	Repair and regeneration of body tissue; constitutes part of all enzymes and hormones such as insulin, adrenalin, and thyroxin; essential to formation of antibodies that combat infection; regulation of water balance and body neutrality (prevents too much acid or alkali in the blood); provides 4 calories per gram.	(Rare in this country.) Reduced resistance to infection; retarded growth and bone development; Kwashiorkor (failure to grow; irritability, apathy, edema, skin and hair changes; liver enlargement; anemia).	Diets too high in protein (e.g., the Atkins Diet over a long period) will tax the liver and kidneys and can lead to bone deterioration via calcium depletion. If protein is obtained from animal sources, the diet is likely to be too high in fat.
	FATS		
Meat and dairy products, vegetable oils, most nuts, mayonnaise, salad dressings, shortening.	Source of energy and major storage of energy; carrier of fat soluble vitamins A, D, E, K; source of essential fatty acids; enhances food flavor; highest satiety value; essential	Rare in this country since only 10 percent of one's calories need come from fat, and only 2 percent from one essential fatty acid (linoleic acid; necessary for cell growth	Because of caloric density, fats are most usual dietary cause of obesity; possible relationship to arteriovascular disease.

BEST SOURCES	FUNCTIONS	DEFICIENCY SYMPTOMS	RISKS OF MEGADOSES
and function; found in vegetable oils).	constituent of membranes of all cell bodies; insulation; cushions internal organs; provides 9 calories per gram.		
CARBOHYDRATES			
The most healthful sources of carbohydrates are whole grains, fruits, and vegetables. Sugar, corn sweeteners, and honey have little or no nutritional value except for calories.	Major source of energy for nervous system and lungs; allows protein to be used for growth and repair of body tissue; source of fiber; aids fat utilization; carries B vitamins; enhances flavor; provides 4 calories per gram.	Persons on diets devoid of carbohydrates develop starvation symptoms: breakdown of body protein; loss of sodium; dehydration; fatigue; loss of energy; ketosis. Sixty to 100 grams per day will prevent these symptoms.	It is difficult to overeat on complex carbohydrates, but too much of certain high fiber foods may prevent absorption of vitamin B₁₂ and some minerals.
VITAMINS			
A			
Liver, eggs, cheese, butter, margarine, yellow, orange or dark green vegetables, and fruits (e.g., carrots, sweet potatoes, broccoli, leafy greens, cantaloupe).	Maintenance of vision in dim light; necessary for growth and reproduction; essential to health of skin and mucous membranes (nose, digestive tract).	Night blindness; growth failure; deterioration of eye tissue; respiratory infections; rough skin; failure of tooth enamel; gastrointestinal disturbance.	Headache; nausea; drowsiness; hair loss; dry skin; diarrhea; dermatitis; weight loss; loss of appetite; joint pain; menstrual irregularity; fatigue; liver damage; bone damage; injury to central nervous system.

*Sources: Brody, Jane. *Jane Brody's Nutrition Book*. New York: Norton, 1981; Guthrie, H. A. *Introductory Nutrition*. St. Louis: Mosby, 1975.

BEST SOURCES	FUNCTIONS	DEFICIENCY SYMPTOMS	RISKS OF MEGADOSES
	VITAMINS		
	D		
Fortified foods, egg yolks, liver, tuna and salmon, and sunlight for fair-skinned persons (dark-skinned persons require it in diet).	Enhances absorption of calcium and phosphorous; assists in formation and maintenance of bones and teeth.	Rickets in children; defects in bone formation in adults that increase likelihood of fractures and muscle spasms (usually an absorption problem rather than a dietary deficiency).	High levels of calcium deposits throughout body that may be mistaken for cancer in adults; kidney stones; defective bone formation; loss of appetite; high blood pressure; high blood cholesterol.
	E		
Vegetable oils; widely found in small amounts in most plant and animal foods.	Protects against oxidation and spoilage of vitamins A and C, and fatty acids in food; essential to utilization of glucose and fatty acids as energy; aids in use of iron and development of red blood cell membranes.	Rarely seen in humans except in premature infants, impairment of fat absorption, or in laboratory experiments. Impairments in animals (e.g., muscular dystrophy; reproductive failure; central nervous system damage; liver degeneration) have not been reproduced in humans.	Possible, but not definitive, relationships to headaches, blurred vision, and fatigue; thrombophlebitis and coronary embolism; breast enlargement and tumors.

K

Food Sources	Function	Deficiency	Side Effects
Green and yellow vegetables, tubers, fruits and seeds; can be synthesized by intestinal bacteria.	Coagulation of blood; maintenance of bone metabolism; release of energy from glucose and fatty acids.	Hemorrhage; loss of calcium (rare); deficiencies usually due to poor absorption, not diet.	No side effects to naturally occurring vitamin K, but synthetic vitamin can produce jaundice and anemia.

B_1 (Thiamine)

Food Sources	Function	Deficiency	Side Effects
Lean pork, whole grains, legumes, fortified cereal products, and nuts.	Necessary for release of energy from carbohydrates; aids the formation of substances involved in transmission of nerve impulses.	Beriberi; loss of appetite; depression and confusion; headache and fatigue; loss of muscle tone, especially in gastrointestinal tract; loss of coordination. Need for thiamin increases as total food intake increases.	The B vitamins work together; an excess of one can cause a deficiency in others.

B_2 (Riboflavin)

Food Sources	Function	Deficiency	Side Effects
Liver, meat, milk and milk products (except for butter), whole grains, and fortified cereal products.	Involved at many levels in metabolism of carbohydrates, protein, and fats and in energy production; involved in formation of red cells and functions of adrenal and thyroid glands.	Inflammation of lips; cracks around the mouth; dry skin; rarely seen outside the laboratory, except among alcoholics.	None known. See Thiamine.

VITAMINS

BEST SOURCES	FUNCTIONS	DEFICIENCY SYMPTOMS	RISKS OF MEGADOSES
Niacin			
Liver, meat, poultry, peanuts, fish, legumes, whole grains, nuts, tuna, eggs, and fortified cereals. Body can convert tryptophan in protein to niacin.	Essential to the release of energy from carbohydrates, fat, and protein, and to the synthesis of protein and other materials needed to maintain all cells in the body.	Pellagra; dermatitis; diarrhea; depression; irritability; headaches; sleeplessness.	Interference with use of energy by heart muscle; reduces ability to utilize fatty acids for energy during exercise; duodenal ulcer; abnormal liver function; increased uric acid; aggravates diabetes.
B_6 (Pyridoxine)			
Meats, liver, whole grains, most vegetables, nuts, bananas, and egg yolks.	Necessary to protein metabolism; aids in use of fats; necessary for production of antibodies and formation of red blood cells; necessary for regulation of nervous system.	Anemia; weakness; irritability; nervousness; insomnia; difficulties in walking; skin disorders; kidney stones; oral contraceptives may lead to mild deficiency and depression; otherwise deficiencies are rare.	May produce metabolic irregularities; prolonged use of larger doses can lead to rebound deficiencies when intake returns to normal.
B_{12} (Cobalamin)			
Found only in animal foods.	Essential for growth, healthy nervous tissue, and normal blood formation; necessary for synthesis of genetic material in cellular reproduction.	Pernicious anemia; found only in strict vegetarians, persons with genetic inability to absorb B_{12}, persons who have had part of stomach removed. Parasitic infection can induce deficiency.	None known.

Folacin

Sources	Functions	Deficiency	Toxicity
Liver, kidney, yeast, mushrooms, orange juice, whole grains, dark-green leafy vegetables, and legumes.	Works with B_{12} in building genetic material; assists in formation of blood cells and hemoglobin.	Anemia; during pregnancy may lead to loss of fetus; oral contraceptives impair absorption and increase requirement.	None known, but body will store it, making megadoses potentially dangerous.

Pantothenic Acid

Sources	Functions	Deficiency	Toxicity
Organ meats, fish, and whole grains are richest sources, but it is widely distributed in plant and animal foods.	Essential to release of energy from fat, protein and carbohydrates; assists in formulation of hormones and substances needed for transmission of nerve impulses.	Can slow metabolic processes and decrease resistance to infection; experimentally induced deficiencies: irritability; muscle cramps; impaired coordination; fatigue; depression; gastrointestinal disturbance; respiratory infections (these have not been found outside the laboratory).	Increases the need for thiamine.

Biotin

Sources	Functions	Deficiency	Toxicity
Liver, kidney, milk, egg yolk, yeast, nuts, and legumes. Some biotin is formed by microorganisms in the intestine.	Aids in synthesis of fatty acids and release of energy from both fats and carbohydrates; involved in protein synthesis.	Dermatitis; loss of hair; muscle deterioration; loss of appetite; nausea; muscle pains.	None known.

VITAMINS

BEST SOURCES	FUNCTIONS	DEFICIENCY SYMPTOMS	RISKS OF MEGADOSES
C (Ascorbic Acid)			
Citrus fruits, tomatoes, strawberries, melon, dark-green vegetables, potatoes, cabbage (raw), and sprouts.	Aids in formation of substance that binds cells together (collagen); promotes healthy bones, teeth, and capillaries; assists in utilization of many other nutrients (e.g., iron, calcium, folacin, protein); may help block action of cancer causing agents in digestive tract.	Scurvy; fatigue; weakness; cramps; shortness of breath; aching bones; skin problems; hemorrhaging of gums; loss of appetite; irritability.	Dependency, resulting in rebound deficiency and signs of scurvy when intake returns to normal; kidney stones; urinary tract irritation; increased blood clotting tendency.

MINERALS

BEST SOURCES	FUNCTIONS	DEFICIENCY SYMPTOMS	RISKS OF MEGADOSES
Calcium			
Milk and milk products (except butter), sardines, salmon with bones, broccoli, green leafy vegetables, and unhulled sesame seeds.	Formation of bones and teeth; maintenance of cell membranes; activation of enzymes.	Abnormal bone growth in children and bone deterioration in adults; danger of fractures.	(Rare) impaired absorption of other minerals; calcium deposits in tissues which may simulate cancer on X ray; fatigue.
Phosphorus			
Meat, fish, eggs, poultry, whole grains, cheese, and legumes.	Formation of bones and teeth; regulates release of energy from fat, protein, and carbohydrates; involved in	Rare except in persons who use antacids excessively; fatigue, loss of appetite; bone loss.	Creates imbalance with calcium and appearance of calcium deficiency.

absorption and transport of other nutrients; synthesis of genetic materials essential to cell reproduction; part of cell membranes and enzymes.

Mineral	Sources	Functions	Deficiency Symptoms	Toxicity / Excess
Magnesium	Green leafy vegetables, nuts, soybeans, and whole grains.	Involved in hundreds of biological reactions: release of energy; protein synthesis; bone formation; nerve impulse conduction; maintenance of normal metabolism; adaptation to cold.	Loss of muscular control; heart beat irregularities; cramps; weaknesses; irritability and nervousness.	Imbalance with calcium leading to disturbance of heart and central nervous system function.
Iron	Liver, red meats, egg yolk, dried fruits, legumes, molasses, whole grains, and greens (collard, kale, mustard, and turnip).	Transport of oxygen in blood; constituent of enzymes and proteins; resistance to infection.	Anemia; easy fatigue; decreased resistance to infection; pallor; shortness of breath.	Toxic build-up in internal organs; bone disease (rare except in persons with inherited defect in iron absorption, or who are overzealous in use of iron supplements).
Potassium	Prunes, dried apricots, bananas, orange juice, meat, milk, salmon, potatoes, peanut butter, tomatoes, molasses, dried beans and peas, and melons.	Release of energy from carbohydrates, protein, and fat; protein synthesis; transmission of nerve impulses; water and electrolyte balance.	Muscle weakness; heart abnormalities; bloating; can be caused by diarrhea, vomiting, use of diuretics, or excessive perspiration.	Heart abnormalities; muscular paralysis.

266 / Appendix B

BEST SOURCES	FUNCTIONS	DEFICIENCY SYMPTOMS	RISKS OF MEGADOSES
MINERALS			
Copper			
Liver, shellfish, nuts, mushrooms, whole grains, cocoa, and cherries.	Facilitates utilization of iron; synthesis of materials coating nerve fibers; part of enzymes involved in protein synthesis and respiration.	Depressed iron absorption; defective red blood cells; demineralization of bone (associated with severe malnutrition).	Diarrhea and vomiting; may occur from cooking acid foods in unlined copper pots.
Zinc			
Meat, fish, eggs, poultry, whole grains, and dairy products.	Aids metabolism of other nutrients; assists in energy and protein metabolism; necessary for action of insulin; aids healing of wounds.	Delayed healing of wounds; loss of appetite and taste sensation; failure to grow in children and abnormal brain development in the fetus.	(Rare) Loss of iron and copper leading to anemia; nausea; vomiting; possible relationship to arteriosclerosis.
Iodine			
Saltwater fish, iodized salt, grains, fruits, and vegetables grown in iodine soil.	Part of thyroid hormones; regulation of growth, development, and metabolic rate.	Goiter; cretinism in newborn children; prolonged deficiency during developmental years can result in poor skin and hair condition.	Not known.
Chromium			
Found almost exclusively in foods of plant origin: vegetables, whole grains, dried beans, peanuts, and yeast.	Utilization of glucose.	Reduced glucose tolerance and possible link to adult-onset diabetes; disturbed protein metabolism.	Not known.

APPENDIX C

Scientific Background

MEASUREMENT OF OBESITY

Height–weight tables, such as the one reproduced in Appendix A, are typically used as guides to average and desirable weight. Although these tables were designed to predict longevity, they are often used to measure obesity. It is assumed that persons who lead sedentary lives and are 20 percent above the weights listed in the table will also have abnormally large quantities of adipose tissue. However, height–weight tables are less than satisfactory since people can be overweight and not obese (football players, weight lifters) and many persons of average weight have a great deal of body fat which may have more implications for health than weight per se. Researchers and clinicians are searching for ways of measuring body fat that will have greater utility for research on health-related issues.

It is possible to measure body fat more directly but much more inconveniently with underwater weighing, emission of radioactive potassium from the body, or inert gas uptake. Many clinicians are beginning to employ estimations made by using calipers to measure the thickness of fat pads at various body sites; others suggest using body circumference measurements (Katch & McArdle, 1977). At the present time, no general standard exists for a judgment of obesity using these methods of measurement (Katahn, 1980). The sex-specific 85th percentile level of the tricepts skinfold thickness for persons age 20–29 was used to evaluate the prevalence of obesity in the United States in one large survey (Bray, 1980, report of the Health and Nutrition Examination Survey 1 by the National Center for Health Statistics). However, fat sites other than the tricepts may have greater health implications. For example, the size of the subscapular skinfold may be more closely related to blood pressure, diabetes, and hypercholesterolemia (Sims, 1980).

Because skinfold measurement requires considerable skill and practice, other approaches which correlate more highly with body fat than simple body weight but require less skill than the use of calipers are being sought. Perhaps the most promising is the body mass index (weight in kilograms divided by height squared in meters). This index has a fairly high correlation with more direct measurement of body fat and is simple to use. West (1980) suggests a standard or "ideal" body mass index for men (22.1) and women (20.6) based on weights without clothes and heights without shoes. It is thus easy to compute the body mass index for any given person as a percentage of standard without using tables. West also points out that waist girth is a simple but good index of fatness that is too little used. Men with a waist girth exceeding thirty-six inches and women with girths greater than thirty inches will almost always be too fat. It seems likely that the body mass index will see the greatest use in the future and authorities may soon come to some agreement on just what percentage above some standard constitutes obesity. Further research will then determine the extent to which deviations in either direction have significant health implications.

DANGERS OF LOW CALORIE DIETING

According to the National Research Council Committee on Recommended Dietary Allowances, care must be exercised in the design of any reducing diet since a reduction in calories increases the difficulty of obtaining recommended allowances of many nutrients, especially calcium, iron, and niacin. In a classic study done by Dr. Ancel Keys and his associates at the University of Minnesota as long ago as 1950, male volunteers on a well-balanced diet except for reduced caloric level (approximately 1570 calories per day), developed serious physical and psychological symptoms over a twenty-four week period. Individuals using the behavior modification approach to modifying faulty eating patterns seem just as likely to suffer from deficient consumption of iron, calcium, niacin, thiamine, and riboflavin as are individuals on any low calorie reducing diet (Ritt, Jordan, & Levitz, 1979).

Low calorie diets decrease body metabolism (Apflebaum, 1975; Garrow, 1978) and make it easier to gain weight on fewer calories than were required prior to dieting. Dyrenforth, Wooley, and Wooley (1980) provide a lucid exposition of the mechanisms involved and explain why, upon the resumption of normal eating, individuals are likely to end up heavier than they were before with a larger percentage of weight in body fat than existed prior to dieting.

There is a great deal of evidence to show that when carbohydrate is not present in the diet in sufficient quantities, the body uses its own lean tissue mass (protein) for energy. This leads to a loss of muscle mass, low energy levels, and, in addition to a further lowering of the basal metabolic

rate, a large water loss as the body works to rid itself of the toxic byproducts of protein metabolism.

VALUE OF A HIGH COMPLEX CARBOHYDRATE DIET

A diet high in complex carbohydrates will be high in nutrients relative
to calories. In addition, it assures adequate dietary fiber of which some
varieties have been shown, in a study done for the U. S. Department of
Agriculture by Drs. Kelsay, Behall, and Prather, to prevent 4.8 percent of
the caloric value of food eaten from being absorbed. An average of 10
grams of additional fat was excreted in the stools of participants in that
study.

Other values of a diet high in complex carbohydrate and dietary fiber
have been summarized in a bulletin by the Institute of Food Technologists'
Expert Panel on Food Safety and Nutrition and the Committee on Public
Information (*Contemporary Nutrition,* 1979). Such diets may be of value in
the prevention and treatment of constipation, diverticulosis, cardiovascular diseases, cancer, diabetes, and weight loss. Specifically, fiber is of value
in relieving constipation because it produces bulkier but soft stools. This
may in turn have some value in preventing hemorrhoids and varicose veins.
Diverticulosis may develop from diets low in fiber and a fiber containing
diet has been shown to cure diverticulosis in rats. In humans, diverticulitis
is now being treated with a high fiber diet with good results. A diet high
in fiber may lower blood cholesterol levels and according to some studies
may provide protection from cancer of the colon and rectum. The panel
reports that in one study blood sugar levels of patients taking insulin were
significantly lower on a high fiber diet (however, diabetics should not change
to a high fiber diet without the advice of a physician). There is also some
evidence from preliminary studies that high fiber diets may be useful in
the promotion of weight loss. For example, high fiber breads frequently
contain fewer calories than standard breads, and they may also lead to a
reduced consumption by increasing a feeling of satiety. However, the panel
also warns that extremely high levels of fiber may cause loss of nutrients
due to the binding of certain minerals to the phytic acid present in certain
plant-based foods. This will not occur if one follows the recommendations
of the Select Committee on Nutrition and Human Needs of the United
States Senate which are incorporated in this book.

The capacity for endurance work can be greatly enhanced by a high
carbohydrate diet (study quoted by Flatt, 1980). According to Flatt, a high
carbohydrate intake relative to fat may lead to a restoration of the body's
glycogen stores after physical activity with fewer total calories ingested. A
high carbohydrate diet may make weight control and dieting much easier
if, as Flatt suggests, the body regulates its total caloric intake closely around

its need for carbohydrate, the nutrient responsible for maintaining the body's glycogen stores.

VALUE OF PHYSICAL ACTIVITY

Led by Dr. Jean Mayer (1968), more and more investigators are paying attention to the value of physical activity in the maintenance of desirable weight. Decreased physical activity, rather than increased consumption of calories, seems to be associated with the development and maintenance of obesity (Van Itallie, 1980).

While some investigators still believe that it may be easier to eat 350 fewer calories per day than to expend that much energy in extra physical activity (Van Itallie, 1980; Garrow, 1978), the fact remains that as many as 95 percent of the people who lose weight by dieting, without attention to increasing activity, will have regained their weight within five years. In a recent study of a group of forty-four massively overweight individuals (averaging 108 pounds above desirable weight), Katahn and his associates (1981) report that only 5 percent were consistently adhering to dietary restriction during a follow-up investigation eighteen months after treatment, but, in contrast, 40 percent were sustaining an activity level averaging 200 calories higher than when they began treatment. All of this latter group of individuals were lighter than when they started their weight reduction program. On the average, this group also maintained all of the weight they had lost during their treatment.

There are many other values to physical conditioning in addition to an increased ability to control one's weight: plasma insulin levels decrease, sensitivity to insulin increases in both adipose and muscle tissue, triglycerides decrease, oxygen consumption in muscles increases, ability to dissolve blood clots increases, stroke volume of the heart increases, the heart rate decreases in response to work, both heart and muscle tissue increase in their capacity to extract oxygen from the blood, and blood pressure is slightly lowered (Van Itallie, 1980). However, sudden increases in physical activity can be dangerous to persons with coronary artery disease and to persons seriously overweight. Proper conditioning is necessary to prevent orthopedic problems.

Further evidence is continuing to appear in the research literature supporting the use of physical activity in the treatment of obesity. At follow-up periods from twenty-four weeks to one year after treatment, exercise has been found to facilitate continued weight loss and maintenance by several investigators (Dahlkoetter, Callahan, & Linton, 1979; Harris & Hallbauer, 1973; Stalonas, Johnson, & Christ, 1978). Leon, Conrad, Hunninghake, and Serfass (1979) report that vigorous walking resulted not only in a reduction of body fat stores, but in reduced endogenous insulin requirements and food intake and may improve the ability to eliminate cholesterol by increasing the plasma high density lipoprotein fraction. Franklin and Rubenfire (1980) recommend exercise for periods greater than twenty or thirty minutes since fat stores are increasingly utilized relative to carbohydrate as exercise progresses. Recognizing the value of exercise in the treatment and prevention of obesity, Jeffrey and Lenmitzer (1981) make specific proposals for increasing good physical activity habits including the establishment of national physical fitness goals, improved physical education programs, expanded employer-sponsored sports facilities and programs, tax incentives, and changes in the focus of school athletic programs in order to encourage each child to develop an interest and enjoyment from physical activity that would last throughout life.

ORIGINS OF OBESITY AND ITS REMEDY

Body composition and weight are influenced by a host of physiological, biochemical, and sociocultural variables, some of which are primarily under the control of genetic factors. Others can be influenced by a person's lifestyle. Three major reviews have recently appeared (Bray, 1980; Stunkard, 1978; Ross Conference on Medical Research, 1980). Rodin (1980) in particular presents an excellent discussion of the neurohormonal basis of obesity and the neurohormonal reactions that occur in response to obesity caused by lifestyle variables. She states (p. 54):

The incidence of obesity seems to be particularly high in populations whose diet is high in fat and whose level of physical activity is low. The trend toward obesity is so pronounced as to suggest that the combined effects of a high fat diet and lifestyle providing for limited physical activity could be synergistic factors in the pathogenesis of obesity.

However, Rodin concludes, agreeing with Garrow (1978), that simple caloric expenditure by exercise may not be the critical, or the main factor, determining energy expenditure or intake in affluent societies. This conclusion is evidently based on the valid observation that the major part of one's caloric needs is generally determined by basal metabolic processes and the amount of additional energy needed in one's work (Garrow, 1978). In affluent societies 99 percent of the work is done by machine rather than by muscle (Balabanski, 1979), which means that few people expend energy much above their resting rates in their occupations. Figuring the average metabolic need at approximately one calorie per kilogram of body weight per hour for a person of average weight (not obese), a 70 kilogram (154 pounds) individual needs approximately 1680 calories to maintain basal metabolic processes in a twenty-four-hour period. If this person requires only an additional 10 percent to perform his work (the amount usually calculated as the difference between basal metabolic rate and resting metabolic rate) because his work is sedentary, *in eight hours he will use only 56 additional calories.* (He might just as well have stayed in bed.) In just one hour of tennis, he would need approximately 400 additional calories; in one hour of jogging at a nine to ten minute pace, he would burn an additional 600 calories. This illustrates that one hour of exercise can easily account for 20 percent of one's total caloric needs. Put another way, 20 percent of one's daily needs can be expended in 4 percent of one's time. The jogger is burning the equivalent of almost 60 pounds of fat per year more than he would have burned sitting still for that hour. Of course, the great majority of people may not care to jog an hour a day, and that amount of exercise is not necessary for weight control in persons slightly to moderately obese. Just walking for 45 minutes more each day, either at work or for recreation, will account for the energy contained in twenty to thirty pounds of fat per year. *Thus, the fact that exercise DOES NOT play a critical role in determining energy expenditure or intake in affluent societies should not be interpreted to mean that it CANNOT!*

While only about 5 percent of the obese appear to have metabolic defects due to thyroid deficiency, other enzymatic, hormonal, and physiological processes can predispose one to obesity. Guthrie (1975) points out that there is great variability in the production of enzymes responsible for fat storage and fat mobilization. The rate of lipogenesis in obese persons may be as much as five times greater than normal. Once fat has been deposited in adipose tissue, primarily as triglycerides, it must be broken down into fatty acids and glycerol (a process known as lipolysis) before it can be used as a source of energy in tissues requiring energy. The obese may have low levels of the fat splitting enzyme responsible for lipolysis. In addition, Guthrie points out that once fat has been deposited in adipose tissue, fat cells will again store fat more readily after it has been removed. Thus, she states, it is easier for a person who has been obese to become obese again than it is for one who has never been overweight. Overweight individuals also vary from normal in their levels of insulin and other endocrine secretions that affect the mobilization of fat and its deposition in various parts of the body.

Extensive discussions of hormonal influences and the variability among individuals in thermogenesis (heat production) and the thermic effect of food can be found in Bray (1975, 1980) and Stunkard (1978).

A great deal of interest has recently been generated by DeLuise, Blackburn, and Flier (1980) who presented evidence that the obese may have fewer sodium-potassium pump units in their red blood cells than the non-obese. There was a 22 percent difference in the number of such units in the obese subjects in comparison with lean controls. Cation-transport activity was similarly reduced. This finding suggests the possibility of decreased thermogenesis in the obese. This relatively lower thermogenesis has already been found in the muscle and fat cells of genetically obese mice (Guernsey & Morishige, 1979). If between 25 and 50 percent of the total energy involved in basal metabolism is used by sodium pump activity, and the obese prove to average about 20 percent greater efficiency, it means an obese person might need from 100 to 200 fewer calories per day to keep the sodium pumps working.

There is also evidence that variability in thermogenesis can result from variation in the amount of "brown fat" present in the body of animals and humans (Rothwell and Stock, 1979). Brown fat burns calories at a rate many, many times greater than that of ordinary fat. Obese individuals may be deficient in brown fat deposits and may not have the same ability as thin individuals to vary the production of brown fat in response to lifestyle influences.

Whatever the contributing factors to obesity that may be operating in the individual case, however, there is still an imbalance between energy intake and energy expenditure in basal metabolism and additional activity that leads to the storage of energy as fat in one's adipose cells. Fat people who are reasonably active obviously need to pay more attention to those factors that lead to an intake of more calories than they would use each day at a lower weight. This generally means lowering their consumption of fat and simple sugars and finding satisfying alternative lower calorie foods, or substituting alternate activities for eating. Fat people who are sedentary, and this group comprises the great majority of overweight people in the United States, may find it more pleasant to discover activities that they can do well and enjoy, and which incidentally burn the excess calories they like to eat that would otherwise be put into their fat stores.

REFERENCES

Apflebaum, M. Influence of level of energy intake on energy expenditure in man: effects of spontaneous intake, experimental starvation, and experimental overeating. In G. A. Bray (ed.) 1975. *Obesity in perspective.* 1975. Washington, D.C.: U. S. Department of Health, Education, and Welfare.

Balanski, L. 1979. Diet and physical performance in the rehabilitation of obesity. *Bibliotheca nutritio et dieta* 27: 33–40.

Bray, G. A. (ed.). 1975. *Obesity in perspective.* Report No. NIH75-708. Washington, D.C.: U. S. Department of Health, Education, and Welfare.

Bray, G. A. (ed.). 1980. *Obesity in America.* Report No. NIH80-359. Washington, D.C.: U. S. Department of Health, Education, and Welfare.

Dahlkoetter, J.; Callahan, E. J.; & Linton, J. 1979. Obesity and the imbalanced energy equation: exercise vs. eating habit change. *Journal of Consulting and Clinical Psychology* 47, 898–905.

DeLuise, M.; Blackburn, G. L.; & Flier, J. S. 1980. Reduced activity of the red-cell sodium-potassium pump in human obesity. *New England Journal of Medicine* 303, 1017–22.

Dyrenforth, S. R.; Wooley, D. W.; & Wooley, S. C. 1980. A woman's body in a man's world: a review of findings on body image and weight control. In J. R. Kaplan (ed.), *A woman's conflict: the special relationship between women and food.* Englewood Cliffs, N.J.: Prentice-Hall.

Flatt, Jean-Pierre. 1980. Energetics of intermediary metabolism. In Ross Conference Report No. 1. *Assessment of Energy Metabolism in Health and Disease.* Columbus, Ohio: Ross Laboratories.

Franklin, B. A., & Rubenfire, M. 1980. Losing weight through exercise. *Journal of American Medical Association* 244, 377–79.

Garrow, J. S. 1978. *Energy balance and obesity in man.* New York: Elsevier/North-Holland Biomedical Press.

Guthrie, H. A. 1975. *Introductory nutrition.* St. Louis: Mosby.

Guernsey, D. L., & Morishige, W. K. 1979. Na^+ pump activity and nuclear T_3 receptors in tissues of genetically obese (ob/ob) mice. *Metabolism* 28, 629–32.

Harris, M. B., & Hallbauer, E. S. 1973. Self-directed weight control through eating and exercise. *Behavior Research and Therapy,* 11, 523–29.

Institute of Food Technologists' Expert Panel on Food Safety and Nutrition and the Committee on Public Information. Dietary fiber. 1979. *Contemporary Nutrition* 4, No. 9.

Jeffrey, D. B., & Lenmitzer, N. 1981. Diet, exercise, obesity, and related mental analysis. In J. M. Ferguson and C. B. Taylor (eds.), *The comprehensive handbook of behavioral medicine,* Vol. 2. Jamaica, NY: Spectrum Publications.

Katahn, M. Obesity. In R. H. Woody (ed.) 1980. *Encyclopedia of clinical assessment.* San Francisco: Jossey-Bass 319–30.

Katahn, M.; Thackrey, M.; Pleas, J.; and Walston, K. 1981. Predicting weight loss and maintenance in massive obesity. Paper presented at the Annual Meeting of the American Public Health Association, Los Angeles.

Katch, F. J., & McArdle, W. D. 1977. *Nutrition, weight control, and exercise.* Boston: Houghton Mifflin.

Leon, A. S.; Conrad, J.; Hunninghake, D. B.; & Serfass, R. 1979. Effects of a vigorous walking program on body composition and carbohydrate and lipid metabolism of obese young men. *American Journal of Clinical Nutrition* 32, 1776–87.

Mayer, J. 1968. *A diet for living.* New York: Pocket Books.

Ritt, R. S.; Jordan, H. A.; & Levitz, L. S. 1979. Changes in nutrient intake during a behavioral weight control program. *Journal of American Dietetic Association* 74, 325–30.

Rodin, J. 1980. Pathogenesis of obesity: energy intake and expenditure. In G. A. Bray (ed.), *Obesity in America*. Washington, D.C.: U. S. Department of Health, Education, and Welfare.

Ross Conference Report No. 1. 1980. *Assessment of energy metabolism in health and disease*. Columbus, Ohio: Ross Laboratories.

Rothwell, N. J.; and Stock, M. J. 1979. A role for brown adipose tissue in diet-induced thermogenesis. *Nature* 281, 31–35.

Sims, E. A. H. 1980. Definitions, criteria, and prevalence of obesity. In G. A. Bray (ed.), *Obesity in America*. Washington, D.C.: U. S. Department of Health, Education, and Welfare.

Stalonas, P. M.; Johnson, W. G.; & Christ, M. 1978. Behavior modification for obesity: the evaluation of exercise, contingency management, and program adherence. *Journal of Consulting and Clinical Psychology* 46, 463–69.

Stunkard, A. J. (ed.). 1978. *Obesity: Basic mechanisms of treatment*. Philadelphia: W. B. Saunders.

Van Itallie, T. B. 1980. Conservative approaches to treatment. In G. A. Bray (ed.), *Obesity in America*. Washington, D.C.: U. S. Department of Health, Education, and Welfare.

West, K. M. 1980. *Obesity in America* (Review). *Annals of Internal Medicine*, 6, 854–55.

BIBLIOGRAPHY

BEHAVIORAL APPROACH TO DIET

Mahoney, M. J., & Mahoney, K. 1976. *Permanent weight control: a total solution to the dieter's dilemma.* New York: Norton.
Stuart, R. B. 1978. *Act thin, stay thin.* New York: Norton.

BICYCLING

Alth, Max. 1972. *All about bikes and bicycling.* New York: Hawthorne.
Balantine, Richard. 1978. *Richard's bicycle book.* New York: Ballantine Books.

GENERAL FITNESS AND NUTRITION

Bailey, Covert. 1978. *Fit or fat.* Boston: Houghton Mifflin.
Brody, J. 1981. *Jane Brody's nutrition book.* New York: Norton.
Cooper, K. 1977. *The aerobics way.* New York: M. Evans.
Katch, F. I., & McArdle, W. D. *Nutrition, weight control, and exercise.* Houghton Mifflin: Boston.
Mayer, Jean. 1977. *A diet for living.* New York: Pocket Books.
Myers, Clayton. 1975. *The official YMCA physical fitness handbook.* New York: Popular Library.
Prudden, Suzy, & Sussman, J. 1978. *Fit for life.* New York: MacMillan.

JOGGING

Donaldson, Rory. 1977. *Guidelines for successful jogging.* Washington, D.C.: National Jogging Association.
Fixx, James. 1977. *The complete book of running.* New York: Random House.
Lance, Kathryn. 1977. *Running for health and beauty: a complete guide for women.* New York: Bobbs-Merrill.

STRENGTH TRAINING

Dobbins, B., & Sprague, K. undated. *The gold's gym weight training book.* Los Angeles: Tarcher.

Schwarzenegger, Arnold. 1979. *Body shaping for women.* New York: Simon and Schuster.

SWIMMING

Lee, Terri. 1978. *Aquacise: water exercises for fitness and figure beauty.* Falls Church, Virginia.

Ryan, Frank. 1978. *Swimming skills.* New York: Penguin.

TENNIS

Gallwey, M. Timothy. 1979. *The inner game of tennis.* New York: Bantam.

Tennis magazine: Instant tennis lessons. 1978. New York: Simon and Schuster.

YOGA

Couch, Jean, & Weaver, Nell. 1980. *Runner's world yoga book.* Mountain View, California: Anderson World.

Hittleman, Richard. 1973. *Yoga: 28 day exercise plan.* New York: Bantam.

SCIENTIFIC BACKGROUND

Bray, G. A. (ed.). 1975. *Obesity in perspective.* Report No. NIH 75-708. Washington, D.C.: U.S. Department of Health, Education, and Welfare.

Bray, G. A. (ed.). 1980. *Obesity in America.* Report No. NIH 80-359. Washington, D.C.: U. S. Department of Health, Education, and Welfare.

Garrow, J. S. 1978. *Energy balance and obesity in man.* New York: Elsevier/North-Holland.

Glasser, William. 1976. *Positive addiction.* New York: Harper & Row.

Guthrie, Helen A. 1979. *Introductory nutrition.* St. Louis: Mosby.

Katahn, M. Obesity. In Woody, R. H. (ed.), 1980. *Encyclopedia of clinical assessment.* San Francisco: Jossey-Bass.

Ross Conference Report No. 1. 1980. *Assessment of energy metabolism in health and disease.* Columbus, Ohio: Ross Laboratories.

Silverstone, J. T. 1975. *Obesity: pathogenesis and management.* Lancaster, England: Medical and Technical Publishing Co.

Stunkard, A. J. (ed.). 1978. *Obesity. basic mechanisms of treatment.* Philadelphia, W. B. Saunders.

WALKING

Calder, Jean. 1977. *Walking: a guide to beautiful walks and trails in America.* New York: William Morrow & Co.

Consumer Guide Editors. 1979. *Complete book of walking.* New York: Simon & Schuster.

Donaldson, Gerald. 1979. *The walking book.* New York: Holt, Rinehart, & Winston.

Dreyfack, Raymond. 1979. *The complete book of walking.* Farnsworth Publishing Co.

Fletcher, Colin. 1976. *The new complete walker: the joys and techniques of hiking and backpacking.* New York: Alfred A. Knopf.

Gale, Bill. 1979. *The wonderful world of walking.* New York: William Morrow & Co.

Kinney Shoe Corporation, & Barnett, Wayne. 1979. *Walking tours of America: mini-tours in major cities on foot.* New York: McMillan.

Man, John. 1979. *Walk! it could change your life.* Paddington Press.

Marchetti, Albert. 1979. *Dr. Marchetti's walking book: getting all the physical benefits of running without taking the risks.* Stein & Day.

Pleas, John. 1981. *Walking is. . .* Nashville: Osaat.

Rudner, Ruth. 1977. *Off and walking: a hiker's guide to American places.* New York: Holt, Rinehart, & Winston.

Strutman, Fred. 1980. *The doctor's walking book.* New York: Ballantine Books.

Sutton, Ann, & Sutton, Myron. 1967. *The Appalachian trail: wilderness on the doorstep.* Philadelphia: J. B. Lippincott.

Xochert, Donald. 1974. *Walking in America.* New York: Alfred A. Knopf.

ABOUT THE AUTHOR

Dr. Martin Katahn, a native of Utica, New York, lives in Nashville, Tennessee, where he is professor of psychology and director of the Weight Management Program at Vanderbilt University.

Dr. Katahn studied the violin under Ivan Galamian at the Juilliard School and toured the country as a first violinist with the Degen String Quartet before taking his doctorate in psychology from Syracuse University.

Once seventy pounds overweight himself, Dr. Katahn now maintains himself at ideal weight through a program of proper nutrition, walking, jogging, and active sports. He has also tested many of the major reducing diets on himself, in order to gauge their physiological and psychological side effects.

Dr. Katahn is the author of over forty scientific articles in professional journals and is a consultant to the Southeastern Region YMCAs in fitness training and weight reduction. He is married and has two children.